Recovery, Renewal, Reclaiming

Recovery, Renewal, Reclaiming:
Anthropological Research toward Healing

Edited by

Lindsey King

Selected Papers from the Annual Meeting of the
Southern Anthropological Society,
Johnson City, Tennessee
March, 2013

Newfound Press
THE UNIVERSITY OF TENNESSEE LIBRARIES, KNOXVILLE

Southern Anthropological Society
Founded 1966

Recovery, Renewal, Reclaiming: Anthropological Research toward Healing
© 2015 by Southern Anthropological Society: southernanthro.org

Print on demand available through University of Tennessee Press.
Digital version: dx.doi.org/10.7290/V74Q7RW4

For all other uses, contact:

Newfound Press
University of Tennessee Libraries
1015 Volunteer Boulevard
Knoxville, TN 37996-1000
newfoundpress.utk.edu

ISBN-13: 978-0-9860803-0-2
ISBN-10: 0-9860803-0-6

Recovery, renewal, reclaiming : anthropological research toward healing / edited by Lindsey King.
   1 online resource (vi, 197 pages) : illustrations -- (Southern Anthropological Society proceedings ; no. 43)
   Includes bibliographical references.
Ethnology -- Southern States -- Congresses. 2. Medical anthropology -- Southern States -- Cross-cultural studies -- Congresses. 3. Public health -- Social aspects -- United States -- Citizen participation -- Case studies -- Congresses. I. King, Lindsey, 1953- editor of compilation. II. Southern Anthropological Society. Meeting (2013 : Johnson City (Tenn.))
   GN560.U6 R43 2015

Book design by Jayne W. Smith
Cover design by C. S. Jenkins

Contents

Introduction   1
Lindsey King

Creating Healthy Community in the Postindustrial City   5
Brian A. Hoey

"The Revolution Will Be Community Grown": Food Justice in the Urban
Agriculture Movement of Detroit   45
James C. Tolleson

Is There a Prescription Drug "Epidemic" in Appalachian Kentucky?:
Media Representations and Implications for Women Who Misuse
Prescription Drugs   85
Lesly-Marie Buer

The Cultural Context of Depression in Appalachia: Evangelical
Christianity and the Experience of Emotional Distress and Healing   117
Susan E. Keefe and Lisa Curtin

Idioms of Distress among White Women Patients at the Southwestern
Lunatic Asylum, Marion, Virginia, 1887-1891   139
Anthony P. Cavender

Water and Cherokee Healing   159
Lisa J. Lefler

The Influences of Vodou on Medical Pluralism and Treatment-Seeking Behavior among Haitian Immigrants in the United States: Suggestions for Cultural Competency Programs   179
Sarah Hoover

Contributors   195

Introduction

Lindsey King

Recovery, renewal, reclaiming; in today's world one cannot peruse the media without finding an illustration of these concepts. Be these stemming from an environmental situation or one that is more personalistic, it cannot be denied that our world is out of balance and that we are engaged in a constant effort to try and regain a healthy equilibrium.

While this situation is not exactly a new one, because of the ease of global communication, it is evident that it is one of our world's biggest worries and challenges. As anthropologists, we are trained to examine cultural situations from several angles, realizing that all aspects of culture are integrated and that in examining these aspects there are many points of view.

In this collection of papers presented at the Southern Anthropological Society 2013 Meeting, hosted by East Tennessee State University in Johnson City, Tennessee, we have an assortment of papers discussing both different types of recovery and the causes that fostered them. We find papers spanning a historical continuum, crossing racial and economic boundaries, and approaching solutions from differing religious and supernatural backgrounds.

The first two chapters focus on landscape and its influence on the health of its people. Brian Hoey, who wrote the opening article, serves as an associate professor at Marshall University, located in

Huntington, West Virginia, a city deemed in 2008 "the unhealthiest city in America." He examines the factors necessary to revitalize the health of urban areas that have been abandoned by the industries that once supported the economic health, if not the physical health, of their cities. Utilizing the definition of landscape as the product of a cultural production of the transformation of the environment, Hoey looks at the history of Huntington and the outmigration of both industry and its residents, resulting in a vista that was not conducive to growth. In this insightful chapter, Hoey relates how the citizens, governing bodies, and businesses of Huntington are turning around both the reputation of their city as well as the relative health of it and its people.

In chapter two, James Tolleson, a graduate of Davidson College, discusses the important issue of food justice. Having previous experience working with programs promoting food justice and health, such as the urban gardening organization Freedom Freedom Growers in Detroit, and working currently with FoodCorps in Greenwood, Mississippi, Tolleson details the racial and economic disproportional access to food that exists in our country. Through his discussion of grassroots programs that provide these populations access to work that can satisfy their need for healthy foods, we learn that agency can indeed be found from the ground up.

The next three chapters have an Appalachian regional focus, examining the use and overuse of prescription drugs in Kentucky, the relationship between evangelical Christianity and depression in Western North Carolina, and the institutionalization of women in the late eighteenth and early nineteenth centuries in southwest Virginia.

Lesly-Marie Buer, a doctoral candidate in anthropology at the University of Kentucky, examines the implications of the local media's framing of drug misuse by women in Appalachia. In particular, she examines what she labels "inflated terminology," such as a drug use "epidemic," which is used by the media to rationalize blighted environment, loss of economic opportunity, and poor health care, rather than examine these aspects as contextual elements that may be factors in the use of these prescription drugs.

Coauthors Susan Keefe and Lisa Curtin, professors of anthropology and psychology respectively at Appalachian State, conducted research with natives of Appalachia diagnosed with depression as well as regional mental health experts and providers on the cultural concepts of depression and its appropriate cultural healing. Building on the findings from 2008 research by Zhang et al., which stated that residents of Appalachia have higher rates of depression and suicide and yet do not show a higher demand for mental health services, Keefe and Curtin examine issues such as depression within the cultural context of evangelical Christianity to help shed light on this discrepancy.

In chapter five, Anthony Cavender, professor of anthropology from East Tennessee State University, examines how diagnosis of mental illness can be culture bound, changing in definition from culture to culture, and also how it may change over time. Through research into the historical records of the Southwestern Lunatic Asylum in Marion, Virginia, between 1887-1891, Cavender reports on the institutionalization of white women, their diagnoses, typical treatments of the period, and how these individual cases represent the Appalachian region within the context of mental health within the United States as a whole.

The last two papers look at examples of medical pluracy and its interconnection to belief systems. In the sixth chapter, medical anthropologist Lisa Lefler, who has worked for many years with the Eastern Band of Cherokee, discusses the importance of water to their worldview. Considering themselves people of water, the Cherokee have culturally constructed rituals that ensure their spiritual, physical, and societal health. In this paper, Lefler considers these traditions and their efficacy through time and related culture change.

In the last chapter, Sarah Hoover, a recent graduate of the master's program in applied medical anthropology from the University of Memphis, investigates complications and misunderstandings that some Haitian immigrants have encountered when seeking health care in the United States. She suggests that physicians who treat these Haitian immigrant populations should seek out cultural competency programs to better understand the societal and religious framework of healing strategies in this culture.

These papers touch upon only a small percentage of research that is being conducted in today's world that focuses on the problems of maintaining health in our world. I hope that in reading the works presented here each of us will be inspired to contribute to solutions that will clear blighted environments, deliver nourishing food to all, ease the lives of marginalized peoples, and lead to respect for all beliefs. With this type of intention, we will be working together to bring balance to our environmental, physical, and spiritual health.

Creating Healthy Community in the Postindustrial City

Brian A. Hoey

Introduction

This chapter explores how community might be reimagined for the benefit of public health as well as to promote incipient social or economic agendas born of progressive citizen action aimed at what is commonly characterized as development or, perhaps, even more broadly as "growth." Can a city like Huntington, West Virginia, emerge as a positive example of what we might term *postindustrial urban regeneration* and perhaps even *community healing*? Can this happen specifically through a grassroots movement now finding local governmental support in a collective attempt to transform this place from one defined primarily by the productive capacity of factories to one that might appeal to small business entrepreneurs—many of whom may be members of a category of potential in-migrants that some scholars, planners and, increasingly, government officials around the United States have called "creatives"? This chapter contributes to academic and popular discussion of how throughout the vast archipelago of former industrial sites—a legacy of a dominative urban-industrial political economy—small cities like Huntington might plan a healthy way forward that promises sustainable, restorative growth in an economic and social landscape that has been shifted by profound structural changes that appear to require a significantly different way of doing things.

Health and Place

Although urban conditions have throughout history presented challenges to health through such factors as crowding, poor diet, and lack of sanitation, widespread industrialization in the nineteenth century greatly exacerbated these longstanding problems. At the same time, emergent large-scale industry added further health risks through rapid, unplanned, and unregulated growth, workplace hazards associated with use of heavy machinery, and exposure to toxic chemicals employed in—as well as pollution from—industrial production. As the negative health impacts of the economic "revolution" became clear by the end of that century, American artists, scholars, health reformers, and community planners came together in an attempt to address mounting concerns. In their deliberations, they pointed not only to *threats* to health associated with urban industry but also to the ability of certain intentionally designed environments to exert potent, restorative, or *therapeutic* influences on states of physical and mental health challenged by ongoing industrial urbanization (Glacken 1967; Hoey 2007; Macy and Bonnemaison 2003).

Specifically, this diverse group of activists sought solutions through approaches that ranged from addressing enduring problems with technical fixes to improve sanitation—a campaign aided by acceptance of an empirically supported "germ theory" of disease—to deliberate allocation of public open space in design plans for new communities. Central figures in the emerging field of landscape architecture, among others, helped frame discussions that would provide both the technical and philosophical underpinnings for principles of urban and regional planning responsible for shaping everyday life in communities of the United States thereafter. Perhaps most notable among them was Frederick Law Olmstead who was not only a designer of New York City's famed Central Park but also served as Secretary General of the United States Sanitary

Commission—a civilian organization that advised the Union Army regarding the physical and mental health of its servicemen during the Civil War.

While for much of the twentieth century economic imperatives dictated how well the design principles that emerged from these early interdisciplinary collaborations would be applied—if at all—the role of environment in public health and civic life is again at the center of merging scholarly and applied interests (cf. R. J. Jackson 2003). Studies in the health sciences have long explored *negative* health effects and risks to at least physical well-being that may be linked to particular locations such as those associated with current or former industrial sites. Beyond this important work, a growing body of research now explores the restorative potential of contact with certain locations through the adopted lens of the *therapeutic landscape* concept. Although its application has been mostly academic in nature and focused on the possibility for *positive* health effects through intimate association with these places (e.g., see Williams 1999; 2007), as defined by the geographer Wilbert Gesler (1996, 96; emphasis added) who first coined the term in the early '90s, the concept could be employed to bring our attention to the "physical and built environments, social conditions, and human perceptions [that] combine to produce an *atmosphere* which is conducive to healing."

The concept of the therapeutic landscape has been criticized for overlooking the importance of everyday places in favor of extraordinary sites of sacred or secular pilgrimage, for example, such as sites of great natural beauty or historical significance. Despite this criticism—or perhaps as a partial answer to it—I have found opportunity within Gesler's original broad conceptualization for a meaningful, everyday application through discussing the importance of *community*—understood as being physical and ideological in nature—for shaping the conditions that contribute to individual and collective health. I am encouraged to consider how community is an *atmosphere,* in Gesler's terms, which we may interpret as a combinative milieu of material and intangible elements within which people must live their lives as both physical and social beings. It bears mentioning that if one such communal atmosphere can serve as a potentially therapeutic agent, it stands to reason that another—for various reasons—may be essentially pathogenic in nature. If there are places—understood as communities—that are health promoting or protective, then there must be places that are variously unhealthy as well. Beliefs, behaviors, and physical conditions characteristic of particular places may contribute to the cause, presentation, and recognition of various forms of ill health and disease.

The concept of therapeutic landscape has become an important theoretical contribution of health geography whose emergence as a field parallels an earlier turn by cultural anthropologists away from a limiting perspective of "place" wherein it is taken as merely the physical space or bare material context within which cultural practices occur. Rejecting the notion that place is a largely neutral setting—a container within which social and cultural life unfolds—ethnographies within the anthropology of health, for example, have for some time presented a dynamic, relational view of physical and mental health. This view holds that human health entails multifaceted interactions between people and their particular biotic, abiotic, and sociocultural environments (e.g., see Devisch 1993; Fadiman 1997; Martin 1994).

As used by anthropologists, such a notion as landscape—whether having therapeutic potential or not—is understood as a cultural production, a symbolic transformation of this environment (cf. J. B. Jackson 1994). Such an understanding takes into account humans, an essentially *anthropogenic* environment, and the manner in which this aggregate atmosphere or milieu is conceptualized, symbolized, produced, and experienced in different places and times (Cosgrove and Daniels 1988; Hirsch and O'Hanlon 1995; Meinig and Jackson 1979). Similarly, landscape is being used in health geography as a metaphor for complex layerings of cultural understandings, history, social structure, and built environment that converge in particular places and times (Kearns and Moon 2002).

More recently, scholarly work in this vein has contributed—though largely indirectly—to a range of local, state, and federal policy initiatives. The United States Centers for Disease Control and Prevention's (CDC) *Healthy Places* is one such program. This program claims to support the "design and development of built environments that promote physical and mental health by encouraging healthy behaviors, quality of life, and social connectedness" (CDC 2006). Given that the program draws on conclusions of the American Planning Association (APA) regarding so-called *smart growth*, we can see explicit recognition of the fact that seemingly mundane planning elements such as zoning—local ordinances that effectively divide a municipality into separate use-designated residential, commercial, and industrial districts—can have a wide-ranging and significant impact on physical and mental health across entire neighborhoods and larger communities (see APA 2002).[1] As a century ago, these contemporary initiatives represent an effort to pair design principles with concern for public health in the broadest possible sense. Of particular significance in programs such as the CDC's *Healthy Places* is a tendency to invoke the decidedly experiential category of "quality of life" as an essential component of the approach to creating healthier places—landscapes that may be thought of as generally therapeutic for those who live and work in them.

One of the first comprehensive studies on the salience of quality of life as a concept for community health and planning was produced by the United States Environmental Protection Agency (EPA) in the early 1970s—only shortly after the agency was established—in order to address environmental degradation and its impact on public health after a century of widespread industrial pollution. The authors described the emerging concept as an attempt to capture "an indefinable measure of society's determination and desire to improve or at least not permit further degradation of its condition." Further, they noted that it should be taken as a way to represent a "yearning of people for something which they feel they have lost or are losing, or have been denied, and which to some extent they wish to regain or acquire." As such, they described it as "a new name for an old notion that refers to the well-being of people . . . as well as to the 'well-being' of the environment in which these people live" (EPA 1972, iii, 1). In my approach to looking at the notion of healthy community, I adopt their insistence on framing quality of life in terms of basic desires or motivations—as well as attending to the well-being of both *people* and the *place* in which they live. As a concept, quality of life relates well to the idea of therapeutic landscape given how—as suggested here in terms of what is described as *yearning*—both address "health seeking behavior." This sort of behavior is something that we may understand as an active quest by people to modify their everyday practices and the environment in which they live and work so as to improve overall health.

A multitude of related disciplines take as a fact that quantitative indicators of health vary across geographic locations. However, etiological explanations within these fields as to *why* we see differences in morbidity (the prevalence of certain diseases in a population) and mortality (death that might result from those diseases in that population) may vary greatly. For the most part, however, those fields concerned with explaining such distributional variation of disease—such as epidemiology—have tended to focus on individual-level risk factors, which are typically seen as associated with such aspects as personal behavior or genetic difference or both. Following this emphasis, differences in the health of particular geographically defined populations may be taken as a direct outcome of presumed "cultural" or "racial" characteristics that—within this approach—are attributed to persons living in a given place. Not surprisingly, social scientists whose interests lie in the area of public health have found such a limited explanatory approach deficient. Generally speaking, these scholars argue that health—especially of socially marginal peoples (e.g., poor and minority groups)—is determined at least as much, if not more, by *structural* conditions that lead to inadequate access to healthy foods, a highly limited capacity to change individual circumstances due to lack of capital (both social and economic), and disproportionate exposure to environmental toxins, than by personal *lifestyles*. They also call attention to the fact that behaviors so seemingly individual in nature as those generally lumped in the category of "lifestyle" are variously enabled or constrained by particular socioeconomic contexts. Only by acknowledging broad structural conditions—sometimes referred to as *upstream* factors in the public health literature—within which people must live their lives can we avoid potentially placing the bulk of responsibility on sufferers themselves for their ill health.

Researchers in disciplines such as anthropology and sociology have brought renewed exploration of the ways in which *context*—understood in a variety of different ways and captured through such broad concepts as landscape, place, or community to which I have already referred—may affect health outcomes (e.g., see Balshem 1993, MacIntyre, MacIver, and Sooman 1993, Robert 1998). Fortunately, such research has not languished in academic journals. We can clearly see the substance of these efforts expressed in a report by a special committee convened by the US Department of Health and Human Services (DHHS). The *Secretary's Advisory Committee on National Health Promotion and Disease Prevention Objectives for 2020* aims to focus a national discussion regarding public health policy initiatives specifically on what the authors characterize as the broad "societal determinants of health" (DHHS 2008, 21).

In the history of Western medicine, it is not as if scholars have only more recently questioned the role of context in shaping the conditions for human health. At least since Hippocrates in the fifth century BCE such readily observable aspects as natural and built environments were considered essential factors in the health of particular populations. Hippocrates is credited with laying the foundation for concepts basic to modern fields of public health and epidemiology in a book titled *On Airs, Waters, and Places*—a principal work within a large corpus attributed to him. When encountering incidences of collective ill health, he encouraged health practitioners to focus their analysis on elements that could be assigned to the following categories: *person* (who is being affected), *place* (where the condition occurs), and *time* (when, or more specifically, over what period, the condition occurs). This basic set of investigative categories has become fundamental to descriptive epidemiological study, which is characterized by a focus on the amount and distribution of disease within a population. I find an allied interest with this field (and its analytic counterpart) in the anthropology of health in that such categories as person, place, and time have long been essential to an ethnographic approach to fieldwork where—when exploring sociocultural phenomenona—the researcher asks a related series of questions: Why do we see these particular people exhibiting a given behavior? What can we determine about how the specific context may influence this observed behavior? What might this point in the history of this place mean for the people involved? These kinds of questions have informed my inquiry into the impact of cultural,

CREATING HEALTHY COMMUNITY

social, and economic factors not only on community health but also the health of community.

Following leads touched on here, envision a strategically inclusive perspective wherein not only physical and mental health of individuals or groups within geographically (as opposed to biologically) defined communities are considered but also the health of communities themselves as such. From this point of view, we could investigate not only the standard quantitative indicators and broad objective measures of health but also the impact played by such taken-for-granted contributing factors as economic and social conditions as well as culturally informed, public perceptions and even how a given community is imagined and represented both within that place by those who live there and externally by others well outside that place. My recent work examines the relationships among these factors in the context of a former industrial city now earnestly attempting—at a variety of levels ranging from the grassroots to the formal—to redefine itself in the twenty-first century. These efforts are already having significant impact on quality of life for its residents.

The Industrial City

Writing in the early twentieth century, the urban historian Lewis Mumford (1925) described the emerging conditions for what he termed a *fourth migration*—the latest in a string of important migratory periods in the United States that began with pioneer settlement. Mumford understood that whatever materialized as America's next migratory act would become the pattern to dominate the twentieth century. In grappling with where residential and commercial development might be going, he forecast a "radical decentralization" of urban economic and social functions that would redistribute population throughout entire regions in a process we now recognize as suburbanization. In his time, Mumford saw remarkable changes in transportation—including especially the automobile's capacity to reshape the physical and social world—as well as remarkable innovations in communication, such as telephone and radio and extensive electrical transmission. He saw these now basic elements of modern life as profoundly distributive and decentralizing agents for the coming age—ultimately making unnecessary a traditional interdependence with others based on geographic proximity.

Although his focus was largely on the technological and structural conditions for emergence of the suburb on a mass scale, Mumford (1925, 130) asserted that these periods of "flow" that he understood to exist in multiple realms from the physical to the ideological were caused by "new wants and necessities and new ideals of life." He saw shifts in basic cultural values as essential to explaining broad societal changes including residential preferences and, ultimately, the locus of economic growth. Following these emergent, culturally informed desires, consumer demand—coupled with well-intentioned policy reactions to urban problems developed during the height of the industrial revolution—drove the process of suburban deconcentration. In a prescient manner, Mumford was gravely concerned that the next leading community form in America would materialize without the thoughtful planning he deemed necessary to avoid broadening and deepening a host of mounting social and environmental problems. Here we see how Mumford lamented missed opportunities during the previous boom (located in American cities) that led to profound societal costs in the form of what we could today call quality of life through disorderly growth, driven by what he suggested was as a reckless element of the presumed "frontier spirit" of America that callously wasted both natural and human resources:

> Homes blocked and crowded by factories; rivers polluted;
> factories and railway yards seizing sites that should have
> been preserved for recreation; inadequate homes, thrown
> together anyhow, for sale anyhow, inhabited anyhow. The
> result was called prosperity in the Census reports, but
> that was because no one tried to strike a balance between
> the private gains and the social losses. (1925, 131)

As noted earlier, though early twentieth-century efforts to address urban health challenges prompted leaders to usher in important regulatory reforms, a combination of factors—including widespread deindustrialization and subsequent job loss—led to massive and relatively hurried outmigration from industrial cities to burgeoning suburbs in the second half of the twentieth century. This had the combined effect of overwhelming efforts to thoughtfully plan these new developments on the one hand and devastating the capacity of many older urban areas to simply keep themselves up on the other. Given that rapid urbanization had been tied to the growth of industrial economies during the previous two centuries, a shift to "offshoring" industrial production, a growing service-based or knowledge economy, and hasty suburbanization within countries like the United States prompted some late-twentieth century scholars to proclaim—or at least theorize—imminent arrival of a condition given the understandable moniker of *post-industrialism*. In the developed world, such a significant alteration in the sectoral location and nature of employment now leads many to forecast far-reaching changes throughout varied domains of everyday life. Some social theorists speak not simply of sectoral transformation—emergence of an economy driven primarily by activities other than manufacturing—but arrival of full-blown "postindustrial society." Following both the agrarian and industrial revolutions that came before, a possible state of postindustrialism suggests yet another period of radical change that may again transform the way that society itself is organized (Hoey 2015).

Thus, in light of economic restructuring that has led to the widespread shuttering of factories, planning and policy discussions in the United States regarding urban and regional development increasingly associate a postindustrial society with a need to develop models for growth founded on principles consistent with imperatives of what some have called the "new economy." This may be seen at least in some novel attempts by those communities most affected by deindustrialization to attract and retain residents as well as economic capital. How will these places encourage or even define "growth" going forward given the fact that the seemingly solid and previously reassuring industrial floor beneath their feet has partly or wholly collapsed? Heretofore, the prevailing approach to encouraging capital investment in many such places has been to cut taxes and provide cheap land and labor in order to attract big industrial employers. Despite diminished returns for their investments, this continues to be the go-to plan for many state politicians all across the United States. An increasing number of local communities must now challenge this "smokestack chasing" strategy—as it is sometimes called—in their own attempts to usher in a postindustrial economy, at least at their level, and assure a minor stake in what some now take as the inevitable emergence of a broader, postindustrial society.

In their efforts, some towns and cities in the northern tier of midwestern and northeastern states that collectively comprise what many refer to as the Rust Belt—a pejorative label applied to conjure images of decaying industrial places from another economic era—have embraced the postindustrial-inflected promises of what is known as "new urbanist" planning and architectural design (Hoey 2007). At the core of planning prescriptions in this approach to community development is a call to create "healthy neighborhoods" defined by

walkable scale, open spaces for public recreation, a range of housing options and businesses in "mixed-use" design, and a "sense of
place" that evokes traditional, human-scale urbanism—something
that garners its practitioners the label "neo-traditionalist" (Duany
and Plater-Zyberk 1992; Calthorpe 1993).

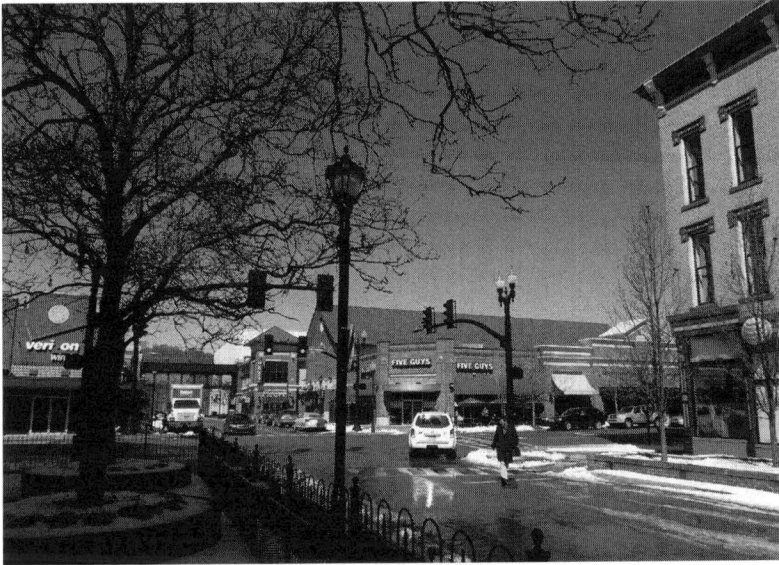

Figure 1. Located in downtown Huntington, Pullman Square is described as a
"lifestyle center." Fashioned in a neotraditional style with elements meant to evoke
the city's railroading heritage, it is located on a tract of land cleared of buildings
in the early 1970s in anticipation of large urban renewal project that only came to
fruition with the opening of the complex in 2004. Photo Credit: Brian A. Hoey.

Proponents of this approach to planning and design assure economic benefit from such development in large part through attracting an emergent social demographic referred to as "cultural creatives"
by sociologist Paul Ray and psychologist Sherry Anderson (2000)
and by urban studies theorist Richard Florida (2004) as the "creative
class." These prognosticators of the postindustrial order ensure that
enduring economic well-being will depend on building the physical

places, shaping the social institutions, and providing the community openness that promote cultural diversity—all of which, they assure, is necessary to invite entrepreneurs of the new economy, accumulate a wealth of human capital, and generate the capacity for future economic innovation. Simply stated, in a postindustrial landscape, such acts are taken as essential for the economic health of communities, and this is itself key to shaping the basic conditions for individual and collective health of the people who live and work there.

Taking a more critical approach, sociologist Sharon Zukin (1990) discusses the potential role of such in-migrants in changing the physical and cultural landscape of the contemporary city through such consumption-driven, identity-seeking forces as expressed in the phenomenon of urban gentrification where low-income residents are displaced by formal or informal projects of urban "renewal." As Japonica Brown-Saracino notes, in virtually all literature on the process of gentrification there is an overwhelming expectation for gentrifiers to possess a "frontier" mentality—akin to that derided by Mumford. They are expected to value places for what they might become rather than what they are either now or have been in the past. They have thus generally been marked as callous opportunists who seek lower-cost housing to build financial capital and status through a transformative process of what might be deemed a kind of self-serving "reclamation" from long-time residents. However, Brown-Saracino's close ethnographic examination at four study sites reveals that a majority of people who appear to fit the category (but not the prevailing stereotype) of "gentrifiers" may more properly belong to a type that she calls the "social preservationists," who she finds "adhere to the preservation ideology and engage in related practices [and] work to preserve the local social ecology" (Brown-Saracino 2009, 9). For former industrial places, the image of a postindustrial society informed by such sensibilities as exhibited by the social preservationist is taken as an ideal to achieve through nurturing investment of such "creative" types for whom growth or community development refers to enhancements in collective quality of life enabled by way of progressively vibrant economic and social environments.

The effort to attract a creative class challenges approaches to encouraging economic investment characterized by smokestack chasing of industries, including those associated with natural resource extraction including coal, gas, oil, and timber. In many places, extant industries such as these and others hold great power because they become—whether real or imagined—essential as providers of jobs who may then dictate planning decisions as well as determine the social and environmental conditions for health within entire regions. Certainly, that is true in the state of West Virginia where coal not only fundamentally reshapes the physical landscape but also purposefully contours—in enduring ways—the political landscape to facilitate extraction of the resource with minimal regulatory constraint (cf. Bell and York 2010).

As a cultural anthropologist, I am prone to engage in an indispensable practice of my discipline, which is to compare cultural practices—at times from disparate contexts—as a way of making the familiar unfamiliar. In this way, in the smokestack chasing of communities all over America, I have come to see a display of belief and behavior akin to Pacific island "cargo cults" documented by my disciplinary colleagues for more than a half-century.[2] The so-called cargo cults of places like Vanuatu are products of great social upheaval among the indigenous peoples of South Pacific islands occupied by US troops during World War II. Apparently awed by an extraordinary ability of American GIs to summon vast amounts of goods like food, clothing, medicine, and weapons through airdrops—from out of the clear blue sky—some islanders developed elaborate systems of belief and ritual practice that mimic elements of military ideologies and behaviors of servicemen that they witnessed, including creating elaborate mock airstrips. As with these cargo cults, to what extent do some local governments hold beliefs and engage in behaviors borrowed from economic models provided by other—comparatively prosperous—communities who have exhibited ability to summon the precious "cargo" of a large employer? In a limited, sometimes desperate, pitch, these places appear to seek what is too often framed as a singular economic salvation through ritualized mimicry where if only they follow the same steps, they too will receive *manna* from an economic heaven.

We get a glimpse of such magical thinking at the community level in an excerpt from my interview with a long-time city planner in Huntington:

> We had been going along as a community through the 1950s with twice the population that we have now. We were feeling pretty good about ourselves. We sat back. The city grew and the private sector drove it. Then all those plants started to go away and everyone was like "Come on, come on back." [*Laughs*] It didn't happen! Then by about 1990, it was pretty clear that they weren't coming back. They're not coming back. It was a slap— we've got to do something. And what is that? The City decided that we were still all about manufacturing so it bought up the old plants and tried to redevelop those grounds. We spent close to 10 million dollars and won the Phoenix Award for brownfield redevelopment. Still, it didn't work. The City felt that it could make its own economic development. Build it and they will come. And we kept at it creating industrial parks without much success. Eventually, it was kind of a desperation move.

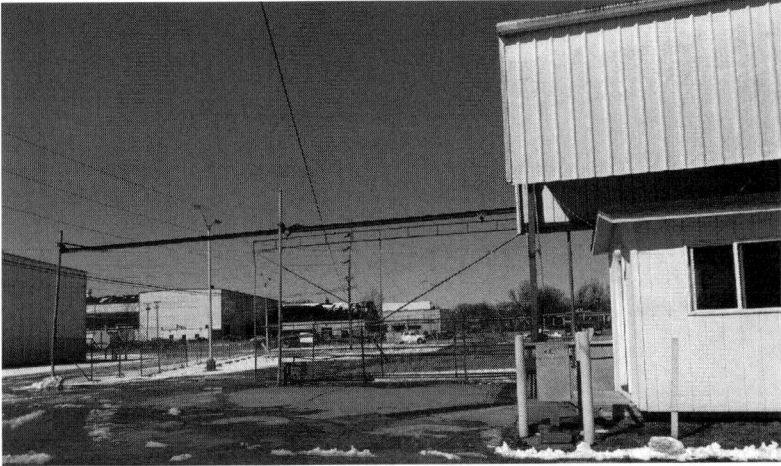

Figure 2. Buildings on the grounds of the former Owens-Illinois Glass Plant redeveloped in the 1990s through efforts of the Huntington Area Development Council and the City of Huntington. Photo Credit: Brian A. Hoey.

Locating Huntington

Huntington, West Virginia, was forged in heavy industry, founded as a key terminal on the Chesapeake and Ohio Railroad in the 1870s. Since reaching its mid-twentieth century peak, today the city's population has been nearly halved by outmigration fostered, in large part, by closure of large industrial employers. Among the relics is the massive ACF Industries plant. Over its history, workers here proudly produced hundreds of thousands of railcars on a sprawling forty-two-acre site beside the Ohio River that now stands unused—a vast, crumbling symbol of the Rust Belt's decline. What would reading this landscape tell us about where this community has been and where it may be going? Following the loss of well-paid industrial jobs, many of the unemployed experience sustained and significant income loss and underemployment. This experience has been shown to significantly increase the likelihood of physical and mental health problems when compared with those who remain continuously employed. At least one study in a community under-going deindustrialization indicated increased mortality even after adjustments were made for background variables such as social class and individual health behaviors or what other studies may term *life-style* (Morris, Cook, and Shaper 1994, 1135).

According to current US Census figures, more than 25 percent of the Huntington's nearly fifty thousand residents live in feder-ally defined conditions of poverty. In what many are prone to call a "vicious cycle," poverty serves to reinforce overall decline and manifests—through interactions with other structural, behavioral, psychosocial, and cultural factors—in individual illness and disease (Robert 1998; cf. Pickett and Pearl 2001). To add insult to years of such injurious deindustrialization, a few years ago the entire com-munity of Huntington was named "the unhealthiest city in America" in popular press headlines based on findings of a CDC survey that found Huntington a national leader in rates of obesity and a dozen other weighty health indicators—measures that include heart dis-ease and diabetes (Stobbe 2008).

This unflattering news attracted attention of celebrity "naked" chef, Jamie Oliver, who then targeted Huntington for a so-called reality TV show, *Jamie Oliver's Food Revolution*, which featured his attempt to get what were often presented as hapless locals eating and behaving more healthily. An especially memorable moment of the series, which came in the premiere episode, was when Oliver con-vinced a local woman to ritualistically inter her deep fryer in the yard while her husband was out of town. Oliver is known for his flamboy-ant style and unapologetic commitment to food prepared in a fresh, unadorned (as in "naked") fashion. The claim that Huntington was the unhealthiest city in America allowed this place and its resi-dents—now framed as a community defined by a particular image and meant to serve as an exemplar of "unhealthy" at the collective level—to serve as perfect foil for Oliver in his effort to promote a "revolutionary" message about diet and lifestyle. Huntington became the purposeful antithesis of the therapeutic landscape. The stage was set, the cameras were rolling, and another social experiment of dramatic outside intervention was—as has been true so many times before—taking place in Appalachia. Attempts to transform the status quo in the region make up a long list of public and private enterprises born of such chronically divergent paths as industrialization and environmental protection, modernization's faith in "progress" and the oft idealized pasts of "heritage" conservation, to the many imaginaries behind a vast range of social, even utopian, experiments from New Deal era intentional communities to New Age communes (cf. Eller 2008; Hicks 2001; Whisnant 1983).

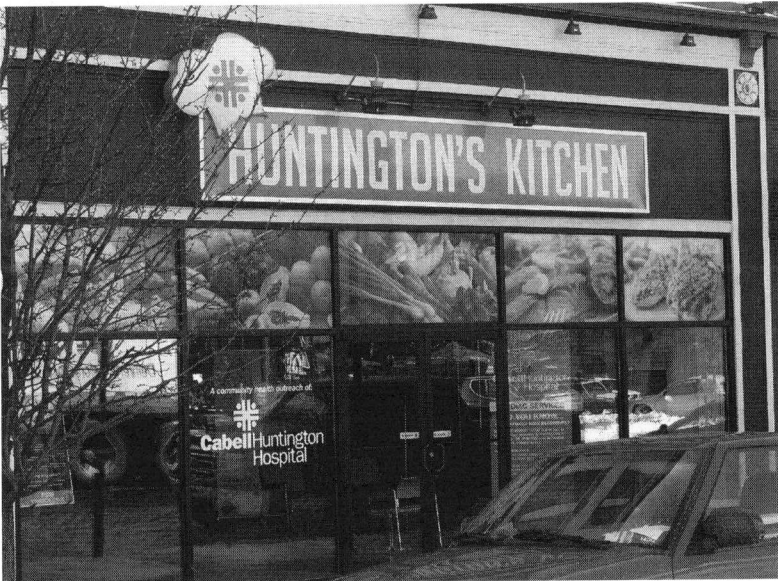

Figure 3. Created for the realty TV series *Jamie Oliver's Food Revolution* in 2010, the former "Jamie's Kitchen" has become "Huntington's Kitchen" and serves the community through ongoing educational programs in cooking, diet and nutrition. Photo Credit: Brian A. Hoey.

In answering a challenge to scholars of Appalachia made at least as early as that by sociologists Alan Banks, Dwight Billings, and Karen Tice (1993, 292) over twenty years ago "to replace unitary notions of Appalachians and Appalachian identity with plural and complexly constructed conceptions of social identity," I seek to offer senses of place emergent in projects of local activists and to detail how these may be variously at odds with popular, stereotypical definitions that prevail beyond the region. In keeping with a respect for what has been called a *critical regionalism* (Powell 2007), I speak not of a sense of place composed of essential qualities imparted by a singular history, set of practices, or a bounded, defined geography, but rather as debate and discourse that variously compete and commingle around the idea or image of community. In this current project, I explore how community—as either real or imagined—may shape the physical or psychosocial conditions that contribute to individual and collective health.

As recognized by Ronald Eller (2008), *defensiveness* can serve as an important part of the process of community building. Specifically, emotional responses by those subject to the harm of popular stereotypes have the power to affect behavior, which may be thought of as depending on deliberate reaction to negative characterization. Clearly, the Associated Press report and subsequent media coverage leading to Jamie Oliver's choice to film an "unscripted" TV series inspired some defensive posturing in the community of Huntington—as was portrayed in the series itself to great narrative effect. More important than on-screen theatrics, however, this behavior appears to have provoked some long-term, critical self-examination and to have produced locally sourced initiatives that aim to present the community in an alternative light—all of which may have lasting, positive impact. While there were already local efforts to address food-related issues, since Oliver's visit, local schools continue to follow many practices introduced during the show's filming.

What was once "Jamie's Kitchen," the main series venue, became "Huntington's Kitchen" and what people now know as a "community food center" as part of the efforts of a local nonprofit medical outreach organization to provide public education for healthy cooking. In addition, the not-for-profit Wild Ramp opened in mid-2012 in the old Baltimore and Ohio train station as a "local food hub" offering direct-from-producer goods to consumers. The hub has done so well that it in mid-2014 it moved to a bigger space located in an area of the community targeted by city government for revitalization. The fruitful initiative to provide year-round access to local produce from small farms was a product of coordinated citizen action and partnerships among recently formed citizen groups such as Create Huntington working together with Huntington's Kitchen as well as Marshall University students completing their senior Capstone projects in my own department. I have come to see these initiatives as rebirth of an earlier movement—discussed below. Today, it is overwhelmingly grassroots and incorporates elements increasingly identifiable as part of a putative postindustrial society.

A Postindustrial City?

In 1993, the Owens-Illinois Glass Plant closed and—as one of the last remaining large industries in Huntington—took with it a staggering 630 mostly well-paying jobs. This single hit increased the city's unemployment rolls by a third. The community was emotionally devastated—it became the proverbial straw that broke the camel's back. Being passive in the face of such loss (really an abandonment) was no longer an option for many residents. In the actions that followed, the desire to prevent further degradation of local conditions was clearly evident—fundamental quality of life was at stake in the community. In an attempt to take control of what appeared a downward spiral, an emergency town meeting was held. Nearly a thousand people attended to discuss ways to stem the community's loss of jobs and, increasingly, its population. Over the next several months, city residents completed a strategic plan guided by three general principles—economic opportunity, sustainable development, and community-based partnerships. Though at least ten years would pass before the substance of this vision would yield lasting results that today promise to transform the community both physically and conceptually, the early '90s movement—dubbed "Our Jobs, Our Children, Our Future" based on a twelve-page special section in the local newspaper—planted a vital seed for thinking about and doing things differently in Huntington.

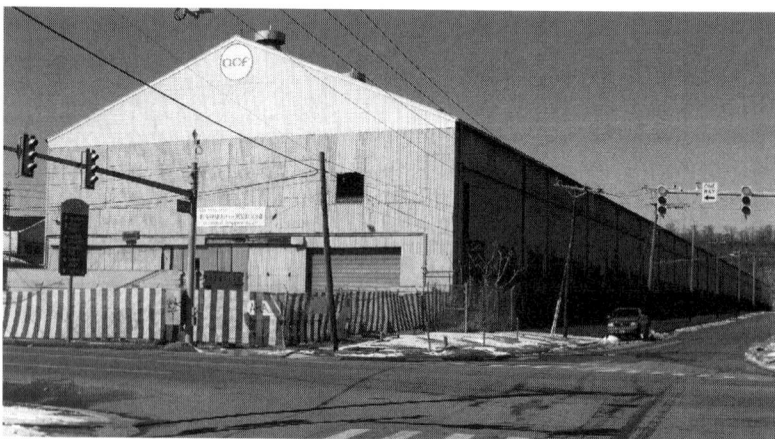

Figure 4. One of many buildings on the abandoned American Car and Foundry (ACF) site in Huntington located on the Ohio River near Marshall University. ACF once employed as many as 1600 people. Photo Credit: Brian A. Hoey.

Today, efforts of increasing numbers of local activists stand in opposition to a range of popular images of the region and in sharp contrast to the Industrial era's dominant order—even while this may not be the case for many of the region's political and economic leaders who seem reluctant to seriously consider alternatives to established ways of "doing business." Despite a recent history of bleak economic conditions and prevailing images of Appalachia as geographically—if not culturally—isolated and thus "backward," Huntington has proved an ideal place to document innovative forms of community building, entrepreneurship, and place marketing according to emerging cultural and economic models that challenge the once dominant paradigm for capital investment.

A legacy of coordinated activism spawn of Owens-Illinois' dramatic closure was picked up in the mid-2000s by the local group that came to be known as Create Huntington. It began in 2006 when then Mayor David Felinton, Marshall University President Dr. Stephen Kopp, and a group of forward-looking citizens came together to discuss ways to address a host of local problems and reenvision Huntington's economic future. Since that time, Create Huntington has evolved into a nonprofit organization wholly dependent on volunteer service, grants, and donations that works to support individual community members and groups in their passionate efforts to improve quality of life in Huntington so that it is an attractive, safe, and diverse community. Among its stated aims, the organization strives to facilitate development and maintenance of a "community vision for progress" and to act so as to "shepherd citizen projects so that progress toward that shared vision is ongoing" while connecting people with the resources and tools as well as individuals and groups that are essential to completing projects collaboratively and efficiently. Most importantly, the organization's mission is to build social capital in the community by strengthening webs of relationships among people who live and work in this place—a connection that enables them to work together in order to improve quality of life through more effective planning and successful completion of projects that fulfill potential in a host of different ways. As noted in the literature for the recent "Create YOUR Huntington" drive by the organization:

> The campaign is about changing the way we think about Huntington and our place in it. It is an acknowledgment that it is time to stop waiting for someone to save our city: a new industry, the government, you name it. They can't save us. It is up to us![3]

Among early influences for the founders of Create Huntington was the first—now annual—CreateWV conference held in 2007. On the morning of my second day of attendance at the second annual conference a year later in 2008, Jeff James—as Chairperson of the Creative Communities team of the public-private partnership known as A Vision Shared that initiated CreateWV—welcomed 395 attendees from across the state and region with a report on the "State of the Creative Community" in West Virginia. In James's address he asserted, "The communities of West Virginia must take ownership of their destiny and embrace the new economy. Otherwise they will end up *downstream* from where others are creating that destiny." I believe that James's use of the term *downstream* was an intended reference to a relative lack of agency or, at least, control. It can be taken, especially in light of recent events, to mean the place that most residents find themselves. This dual meaning works well to describe the reality of life in the state both metaphorically and physically. Downstream describes the location of many of the state's residents at the receiving end, not of any measure of the *affluence* obtained through extractive exploitation of the state's and region's natural and human resources, but rather its considerable *effluence*—a position to which I will return shortly.[5]

Through their actions, "creative" activists such as those who come to the CreateWV conferences each year challenge not only widespread perception of the region and its residents, among other things, as "backward," but also general assumptions of a literature on place and place-attachment. Especially in the case of Appalachia, this literature has emphasized identity defining connections of people to land based on often highly idealized narratives that testify to continuity of familial residency, personal memories, detailed knowledge of the past, and intimate experience in the present. Virtually no attention is given to importance of *future visions* as a dimension in individual or collective sense of place.[4] My assertion is that what is called place making involves acts of both remembering and *imagining*. Specifically, I hold that place image has real consequences for everyday life and well-being. It is the means through which what is imagined—whether out of hope or fear—can become real (Hoey 2010). Images, including the stereotypical, can become reputation and may lead to real-world changes that can be either therapeutic (i.e., health promoting or protective) or pathogenic (i.e., harmful) in terms of individual and communal health.

Here we have a case where place-based identity is shaped through purposeful construction of future visions. Looking at efforts of local activists in Huntington engaged with citizen projects originating through participation in the Create Huntington group provides an opportunity to examine efforts to critically redefine place image both outwardly and inwardly. This redefinition is proceeding, with growing cooperation from local authorities, through purposeful engagement with such trends as "smart growth" and "mixed-use" development expressed in so-called neotraditionalism of New Urbanism as well as other prescriptive approaches believed essential to staking a claim in the landscape of a postindustrial economy.

Reflecting on a recent shift in governmental strategy, Huntington's longtime city planner commented:

> Today the City has learned its lesson, I think. Now we work together with the private sector and local citizens. We do our part by changing the environment—whether that be something as simple as traffic patterns or doing things to improve how people perceive the community. What can we do to attract people who want to live here? We are pursuing "green" initiatives and enhancing our amenities to make our city look more progressive not only to businesses but also potential employees.

Indeed, this is an approach for which there is research-based support. As noted by geographer Alexander Vias (1999), in an emerging economic landscape based on principles of "flexibility," jobs increasingly follow people. In addition to benefits imagined for existing residents, these efforts are a conscious attempt by activists and city government working with receptive local agencies including, the local Convention and Visitors Bureau in Huntington, to woo creatives who pursue lifestyle choices that emphasize the quality of life and "livability" of a community.

Topophilia or Topophobia?

I have conducted considerable research to support my assertion that employers and workers within specific sectors of the economy are especially sensitive to quality-of-life considerations when making location or relocation decisions (Hoey 2014). Many are within what we now refer to as the knowledge-based area of the economy and associated with emergence of a postindustrial society. Among them are businesses with normally higher-paying jobs than those of other sectors and the capacity to stimulate vigorous, diverse local economies.

As my ongoing research in the American Midwest has shown, competition is strong among towns and cities to attract both these existing businesses as well as talented workers. At the same time, free-agent entrepreneurs looking to start small businesses are increasingly able to locate to geographic areas of their own choosing. In their decision making, quality-of-life considerations weigh heavy. Among the indicators upon which individual or collective migrants (i.e., business entities) base their decisions are an affordable, quality housing stock that retains value, natural amenities such as access to forests, lakes, and rivers, as well as vibrant socially and economically diverse communities that afford ample opportunities for arts and entertainment. In addition, potential migrants weigh issues of health and safety, including the impact of past or ongoing industrial pollution.

When reference is made to *upstream* factors in the public health literature, as I noted earlier, it is typically to a range of structural conditions that may contribute significantly to individual and collective health. Unlike what is considered lifestyle, for example, these conditions should be understood as largely beyond the control of affected persons given entrenched patterns of political and economic power that help to establish and maintain that situation. In a timely and wholly unfortunate illustration of how—in a very real way—such upstream factors impact health, on January 10, 2014, a chemical spill from a Freedom Industries "tank farm" along the Elk River in Charleston, West Virginia, polluted the water supply for some three hundred thousand people in nine counties. The spill became national news for several weeks. West Virginia American Water, the private water utility, has their intake pipe just over a mile downstream from the inadequately prepared facility, which served the coal industry.

The long-term impact on human health due to exposure to the contaminated water is unknown owing to a scarcity of reliable information on the substances involved—something that is regrettably true for many commonly used industrial chemicals. The psychological and economic impacts, however, are immediately demonstrable. Lingering foul taste and sickening odor left residents afraid to drink their water. Businesses were forced to close for weeks at a time or to rely on bottled water for their cooking and cleaning. Visitors question plans to come to the area. Long dubbed and even celebrated as the "Chemical Valley," the most densely populated area of the state may now find this an unfortunate matter of branding in light of national attention connected to the spill. As if this were not enough toxic news attention, as the eager spotlight was shining on state and government officials who twisted themselves in knots through a simultaneous attempt to appease angry citizens by promising that *something* would be done, to assure anxious industry that the *status quo* would not be unduly upset, and to appear willing to address obviously lax regulatory oversight, over one hundred thousand gallons of coal slurry was released into another nearby tributary of the Ohio River. In this instance, the accountable corporate entity is Patriot Coal. In the wake of the Freedom and Patriot spills, there is significant chatter in local and national news reports, personal blogs, and (of course) Facebook about a possible "chemical brain drain" in the state. West Virginia can hardly afford the loss of well-educated talent given that, according to current census data, we are already at the bottom of a list of states indicating residents with at least a bachelor's degree.

Local entrepreneurs—some of whom have been central to efforts to improve quality of life in Huntington and other parts of the state—now wonder whether they can remain comfortable with what lies, ominously, upstream. After all, it has become clear that this is where the real power to affect the health of communities in this state has always been. As noted by the director of the West Virginia Center on

Budget and Policy, Ted Boettner, if the state wants to "attract people here and keep people here, it makes it very difficult if we can't even provide safe water" (quoted in Ward 2014). I have to agree with this simple assessment that ours could become more a landscape of fear than a therapeutic landscape.

As I suggested earlier, we may think of different places as existing on a continuum from the potentially therapeutic to the essentially pathogenic. A therapeutic landscape necessarily represents only one dimension of our relationship with place or, in this case, what geographer Yi-fu Tuan (1974) referred to as *topophilia* as the basis for positive affective attachment between person and place born of comfort and subjective well-being. A landscape of fear—what Tuan (1979) described by way of his notion of *topophobia*—establishes an essentially negative, or at least ambivalent, relationship between people and place that may ultimately induce anxiety, dread, and depression. In her work on the emotional development of children, in particular, Louise Chawla (1992) suggests that the places we inhabit, at all times, have the potential for either light or darkness as there is always a "shadow side" to our relationship. While Chawla's concept evokes the relative darkness, it nevertheless opens the possibility of change in our relationship to any given place. That is to say, this relationship is dynamic. Given recent history in West Virginia, we need to concentrate on banishing the shadows of harmful practices by making way for the light of new opportunities.

Conclusion

While, on the one hand, the shift from heavy industry in the city of Huntington may be framed as a positive development when weighed purely by means of objective measures of health in that closure of factories removes local sources of pollution—even while leaving behind potentially toxic "brownfield" areas that require remediation—on the other hand, the impact of widespread job loss and outmigration is clearly negative. Rising unemployment and outmigration both contribute substantially to deteriorating economic and social conditions. Of the many costs associated with loss of the city's industrial base, we can point to the most obvious loss of jobs, but we must also follow the effect of job loss to the forfeiture of homes and health care, reductions in the tax base—that lead to cuts in essential public services—increases in crime, suicide, drug and alcohol abuse, family violence and depression, declines in cultural resources such as communal organizations, and eventual loss of public faith in civic institutions. While Huntington has done better than many similar places in addressing the impact, the city and its citizens still face ongoing challenges. As time passes, not only does physical infrastructure crumble in the absence of sufficient public revenue, but the very sense of worth and well-being of a place and its people can be fundamentally injured. It becomes extraordinarily difficult for a community to recover from such long-term physical and emotional damage. The effects of deindustrialization can undermine the social fabric of communities. Especially in those places that rely on just one or two industries, it can undermine a community's character and sense of competence.

In many cases, it comes down to a critical reexamination of long-held sources of identity for a community. This may require a sustained, collective effort on the part of a large number of residents to actively redefine themselves. This may be in opposition to a prevailing stereotype that adheres to one of a number of different labels. Here in Huntington, people are faced with the need to challenge images of decline and decay associated with being in the Rust Belt—not to mention the recent stigma adhering to its position downstream to the Chemical Valley spill. The community may be similarly burdened with popular images of Appalachia that are reinforced through sensationalized media representations such as those portrayed in Jamie Oliver's production or, most offensively, in the recent MTV-produced *Buck Wild* television series, which claimed to be an "authentic comedic series following an outrageous group of childhood friends from the rural foothills of West Virginia who love to dodge grown-up responsibilities and always live life with the carefree motto, 'whatever happens, happens.'"[5] In light of media attention after the recent spills, it seems that many Americans may now have the sense that in West Virginia, similarly irresponsible business leaders do what they please in the name of shortsighted profit and that, indeed, whatever happens downstream, simply happens. Finally, no label is more unambiguously unhealthy as "unhealthiest." This is unless such labels can motivate meaningful, effective action at the individual and collective levels—perhaps through what we might characterize as a *self-critical* defensiveness. Indeed, that is something that I have observed in Huntington over the past several years. Recent events, however, remind us that local efforts to create healthy community can be undone by what goes on just upstream.

In preparing an earlier version of this chapter, I was struck by prerelease news coverage of a comprehensive report from the United States Institute of Medicine, which compares health here to other wealthy countries. It is tellingly subtitled "Shorter Lives, Poorer Health." Upon examination of the final report, I was taken by one of the more remarkable findings: Researchers found *geography* the strongest predictive and protective factor for rising morbidity and mortality even when factoring out differences in wealth, education, and behavior. What should we conclude based on such a stunning finding? Could this suggest that place—the culturally informed milieu in which people live their lives—matters to a degree largely unappreciated outside of the literature I have referenced in this chapter? Based on their findings, the report's authors assert that "meaningful health improvement efforts must extend beyond a focus on health care delivery and include stronger policies affecting health behaviors and the social and environmental determinants of health" (Woolf and Lauden 2013). For my part, I find support in this report for what I have suggested needs to be a fundamental shift from the traditional view of health to one where our towns and cities treat health as a collective *asset* that must involve consideration of *quality of life* as we broaden our attention to include self-defining images of community that can prove to be either harmful or therapeutic. Let us not forget that these images are, at least partly, the combinative result of our own actions and the perceptions that others—perhaps well outside our communities—have of the priorities and values that they associate with these actions.

Thinking in terms suggested by the therapeutic landscape concept, we are encouraged to consider how the physical environment, social conditions, and the ways in which people perceive themselves, others, and the places in which they live and work contribute to an atmosphere that can support health or provoke disease. From a practical point of view, this suggests public policy that goes beyond limited, standardized measures of health born of quantitative data alone. Health is a product of complex interactions of people with their social, cultural, and material environments. I propose that we reimagine community as a place—or a "landscape" in the sense described earlier—in order to promote meaningful changes that impact individual and collective well-being. Recognizing the fundamental importance of a sustainable, diversified local economy for providing opportunities for meaningful, remunerative work, community members as well as leaders must be engaged in the process of exploring new economic models for development that support small-scale, locally initiated entrepreneurialism as opposed to the smokestack chasing of another era. Such a rethinking may be necessary to overcome the health burden borne by former industrial places where today's generation inherits a legacy of environmental toxins, patterns of economic dependency, and stereotyped, limiting labels.

Notes

1. Today's zoning laws are the product of planning responses to the spread of infectious disease associated with high-density residential areas in the nineteenth century as well as with a desire to physically separate potentially harmful places of business and, specifically industrial production, from homes, schools, and places of recreation. The establishment of distinct "zones," together with both widespread car ownership and the development of an extensive system of highways in the mid-twentieth century, encouraged low-density development outside of urban cores. Essentially, zoning is used to designate what areas within a community are "appropriate" for certain, specified uses. Aside from determining what can be developed in a given place, zoning laws can determine how any designated use can be developed through defining such things as densities, building size, and lot coverage.

2. In preparing this chapter, I was encouraged that sociologist Helen Lewis (2007) also described these similarities in her consideration of community development in Appalachia—whether urban or rural.

3. The Create Huntington website (http://www.createhuntington. org) has recently been updated and no longer includes the material quoted here. This material was captured from the website in July 2013.

4. See Wagner 1999 for an exception.

5. I would like to credit this play on words to Merton Rivers with whom I had worked during several canoe expeditions in the area of Millinocket, Maine, during the late 1980s. The aptly named Rivers rented canoes and supplies practically in the shadow of the Great Northern Paper mill that gave rise to the town a century ago. In 2008, the mill closed leaving Millinocket economically decimated

and with the very real challenge of being geographically isolated in the Northern woods. While many local leaders and residents look again to industry others seek alternatives. Having been almost entirely dependent on the mill for providing well-paying jobs for generations, the community has no easy way forward.

6. See the MTV series website at http://www.mtv.com/shows/buckwild/series.jhtml.

Works Cited

APA (American Planning Association). 2002. *Policy Guide on Smart Growth*. http://www.planning.org/policy/guides/adopted/smartgrowth.htm.

Balshem, Martha Levittan. 1993. *Cancer in the Community: Class and Medical Authority, Smithsonian Series in Ethnographic Inquiry*. Washington: Smithsonian Institution Press.

Banks, Alan, Dwight Billings, and Karen Tice. 1993. "Appalachian Studies, Resistance, and Postmodernism." In *Fighting Back in Appalachia: Traditions of Resistance and Change*, edited by S. L. Fisher, 283-301. Philadelphia: Temple University Press.

Bell, Shannon Elizabeth, and Richard York. 2010. "Community Economic Identity: The Coal Industry and Ideology Construction in West Virginia." *Rural Sociology* 75 (1): 111-43.

Brown-Saracino, Japonica. 2009. *A Neighborhood That Never Changes: Gentrification, Social Preservation, and the Search for Authenticity, Fieldwork Encounters and Discoveries*. Chicago: University of Chicago Press.

Calthorpe, Peter. 1993. *The Next American Metropolis: Ecology, Community, and the American Dream*. New York: Princeton Architectural Press.

CDC (Centers for Disease Control and Prevention). 2006. "Health Protection Goals: Criteria and Objectives," Office of Strategy and Innovation. Updated October 4. http://www.cdc.gov/about/goals/default.htm.

Chawla, Louise. "Childhood Place Attachments." In *Place Attachment*, edited by Irwin Altman and Setha Low, 12, 63-86: Springer, 1992.

Cosgrove, Dennis E., and Stephen Daniels. 1988. *The Iconography of Landscape: Essays on the Symbolic Representation, Design, and Use of Past Environments.* New York: Cambridge University Press.

Devisch, Renaat. 1993. *Weaving the Threads of Life: The Khita Gyn-eco-logical Healing Cult among the Yaka.* Chicago: University of Chicago Press.

DHHS (Department of Health and Human Services). 2008. *Phase I Report: The Secretary's Advisory Committee on National Health Promotion and Disease Prevention Objectives for 2020.* Washington, DC: US Government Printing Office.

Duany, Andres, and Elizabeth Plater-Zyberk. 1992. "The Second Coming of the American Small Town." *Wilson Quarterly* 16:19-32.

Eller, Ronald D. 2008. *Uneven Ground: Appalachia since 1945.* Lexington: University Press of Kentucky.

EPA (Environmental Protection Agency). 1972. "The Quality of Life Concept: a Potential New Tool for Decision-Makers." Environmental Studies Division Environmental Protection Agency, Washington, DC: US Government Printing Office.

Fadiman, Anne. 1997. *The Spirit Catches You and You Fall Down: A Hmong Child, Her American Doctors, and the Collision of Two Cultures.* New York: Farrar, Straus, and Giroux.

Florida, Richard L. 2004. *The Rise of the Creative Class and How It's Transforming Work, Leisure, Community and Everyday Life.* New York: Basic Books.

Gesler, William. 1996. "Lourdes: Healing in a Place of Pilgrimage." *Health & Place* 2:95-105.

Glacken, C. 1967. *Traces on the Rhodian Shore: Nature and Culture in Western Thought from Ancient Times to the End of the 18th Century.* Berkeley: University of California Press.

Hicks, George L. 2001. *Experimental Americans: Celo and Utopian Community in the Twentieth Century*. Urbana: University of Illinois Press.

Hirsch, Eric, and Michael O'Hanlon. 1995. *The Anthropology of Landscape: Perspectives on Place and Space*. New York: Oxford University Press.

Hoey, Brian A. 2007. "Therapeutic Uses of Place in the Intentional Space of Community." In *Therapeutic Landscapes*, edited by A. Williams, 297-314. Geographies of Health. Hampshire, England: Ashgate.

———. 2010. "Place for Personhood: Individual and Local Character in Lifestyle Migration." *City & Society* 22:237-61.

———. 2014. *Opting for Elsewhere: Lifestyle Migration in the American Middle Class*. Nashville, TN: Vanderbilt University Press.

———. 2015. Postindustrial Societies. In *International Encyclopedia of the Social and Behavioral Sciences*, edited by Dominic Boyer and Ulf Hannerz. Oxford, England: Elsevier.

Jackson, John Brinckerhoff. 1994. *A Sense of Place, a Sense of Time*. New Haven: Yale University Press.

Jackson, Richard J. 2003. "The Impact of the Built Environment on Health: An Emerging Field." *American Journal of Public Health* 93 (9): 1382-84.

Kearns, Robin A., and G. Moon. 2002. "From Medical to Health Geography: Novelty, Place and Theory after a Decade of Change." *Progress in Human Geography* 26:605-25.

Lewis, Helen Matthews. 2007. "Rebuilding Communities: A 12-Step Recovery Program." *Appalachian Journal* 34:316-25.

MacIntyre, Sally, Sheila MacIver, and Anne Sooman. 1993. "Area, Class and Health: Should We Be Focusing on Places or People? *Journal of Social Policy* 22:213-34.

Macy, Christine, and Sarah Bonnemaison. 2003. *Architecture and Nature Creating the American Landscape*. New York: Routledge.

Martin, Emily. 1994. *Flexible Bodies: Tracking Immunity in American Culture from the Days of Polio to the Age of AIDS*. Boston: Beacon Press.

Meinig, D. W., and John Brinckerhoff Jackson. 1979. *The Interpretation of Ordinary Landscapes: Geographical Essays*. New York: Oxford University Press.

Morris, Joan K., Derek G. Cook, and A. Gerald Shaper. 1994. "Loss of Employment and Mortality." *British Medical Journal* 308 (6937): 1135-39.

Mumford, Lewis. 1925. "The Fourth Migration." *Survey Graphic* 7:130-33.

Pickett, Kate E, and Michelle Pearl. 2001. "Multilevel Analyses of Neighbourhood Socioeconomic Context and Health Outcomes: A Critical Review." *Journal of Epidemiology and Community Health* 55 (2): 111-22.

Powell, Douglas Reichert. 2007. *Critical Regionalism: Connecting Politics and Culture in the American Landscape*. Chapel Hill: University of North Carolina Press.

Ray, Paul H., and Sherry R. Anderson. 2000. *The Cultural Creatives: How 50 Million People Are Changing the World*. New York: Three Rivers Press.

Robert, Stephanie A. 1998. "Community-level Socioeconomic Status Effects on Adult Health." *Journal of Health and Social Behavior* 39 (1): 18-37.

Stobbe, Mike. 2008. "W. Virginia Town Shrugs at Poorest Health Ranking." In *AP Wire Report*. New York: Associated Press.

Tuan, Yi-fu. 1974. *Topophilia: A Study of Environmental Perception, Attitudes, and Values*. Englewood Cliffs, NJ: Prentice-Hall.

———. 1979. *Landscapes of Fear*. Minneapolis: University of Minnesota Press.

Vias, Alexander C. 1999. "Jobs Follow People in the Rural Rocky Mountain West." *Rural Development Perspectives* 14:14-23.

Wagner, Melinda B. 1999. "Measuring Cultural Attachment to Place in a Proposed Power Line Corridor." *Journal of Appalachian Studies* 5 (2): 241-46.

Ward, Ken. 2014. "Patriot Cited Again in Slurry Spill." *Charleston Gazette*, February 21, 2014.

Whisnant, David E. 1983. *All That Is Native and Fine: The Politics of Culture in an American Region*. Chapel Hill: University of North Carolina Press.

Williams, Allison. 1999. *Therapeutic Landscapes: The Dynamic between Place and Wellness*. Lanham, MD: University Press of America.

———. 2007. *Therapeutic Landscapes*. Aldershot, England: Ashgate.

Woolf, Steven H., and Aron Laudan. 2013. "U. S. Health in International Perspective: Shorter Lives, Poorer Health." Washington, DC: National Academies Press.

Zukin, Sharon. 1990. "Socio-spatial Prototypes of a New Organization of Consumption: The Role of Real Cultural Capital." *Sociology* 24 (1): 37-56.

"The Revolution Will Be Community Grown": Food Justice in the Urban Agriculture Movement of Detroit

James C. Tolleson

> What is going to happen to cities like Detroit, which was once the "arsenal of democracy," and others whose apex was tied to manufacturing? Now that they've been abandoned by industry, are we just going to throw them away? Or can we rebuild, redefine, and respirit them as models of twenty-first-century self-reliant and sustainable multicultural communities?
> —Grace Lee Boggs, *The Next American Revolution*

In recent years, Detroit, Michigan, has become a national and international focal point for urban agriculture. While the city works to address the effects of its decades-long economic decline, some have named Detroit a potential model for cities dealing with parallel issues of deindustrialization and joblessness (Runk 2010). However, some Detroiters are concerned about the direction of urban revitalization. In this predominantly African American city, many residents are the descendants of migrants from the rural US South and have known family and community gardens for generations. However, during the summer of 2012, plans for a large agricultural project called "Hantz Farm" prompted Detroit food activist Malik Yakini (2012b) and others to ask the question, "What kind of urban farming will Detroit have?" Yakini and other members of the Detroit Black Community Food Security Network (DBCFSN) challenged the Hantz Farm project, which aimed to purchase over two thousand vacant lots on the east side of Detroit to establish a ten-thousand-acre private farm with the express purpose of creating "land scarcity" (Holt-Giménez 2011; Dolan 2012). The Hantz Farm controversy offered an opportunity to highlight the vision of food justice activists with a different plan for urban agriculture and rebuilding Detroit, one based on grassroots development and alternative economic structures built by and for historically oppressed Detroit residents.

When I began looking at the different organizations involved in urban agriculture in Detroit, I focused on the Feedom Freedom Growers (FFG), a small family-based organization associated with the Detroit Black Community Food Security Network. During the limited time (eight weeks) that I spent with the FFG conducting interviews, participant observations, and document collection, I started with two primary questions: (1) How is the food justice activism of the FFG influenced by traditions within the Black Freedom Movement? (2) What is the role of community building in the FFG's work?

Early on, I was intrigued by how one of the cofounders, Wayne, described his experiences as a member of the Black Panther Party (BPP) in the 1970s. He frequently referenced the BPP in relation to his current work with the FFG. Due to his leadership in the FFG, Wayne's experiences with the BPP and other facets of Black Freedom Movements were a strong influence on many FFG participants. In this paper, I identify several ways that the BPP influences the work of the FFG and discuss the significance of this influence for food justice activism.

Another early observation was that members of the FFG often mentioned community and community building in descriptions of their work, including building relationships with neighbors and using a communal or collective process for liberation. I wanted to understand where this tendency to focus on community building came from and, again, what it meant for food justice activism.

In the following sections, I will provide a historical backdrop for the food insecurity that exists in Detroit today and discuss the perspectives of the FFG's farmers, activists, and educators in relation to the concept of *food justice*, a term used to describe food activism arising largely out of communities of color and in contrast to some of the norms within the mostly white, middle-class dominant food movement (Alkon and Agyeman 2011). *Food justice*, while a relatively new term in academic and activist work, describes food activism that uplifts the issues of equity and justice that often get marginalized in the dominant food and environmental movements. The food justice elements of the urban agriculture movement in Detroit articulate the need for a historically and culturally rooted social movement, a grassroots approach to engaging community members in a collective manner to solve problems, reclaiming land from public and private entities who do not use the land for common benefit, and new ways of measuring justice and sustainability in development.

Detroit: Motor City to "Food Desert"?

On July 18, 2013, the city of Detroit, Michigan, hit front-page news around the world for verging on "the nation's largest public sector bankruptcy" (Isidore 2013; Maynard 2013; Rushe 2013). Several prominent Detroiters responded, including City Councilmember JoAnn Watson (2013), who wrote an article entitled "THE CITY OF DETROIT HAS NOT FILED BANKRUPTCY!" in which she explained that Michigan Governor Rick Snyder had actually been the one to file bankruptcy via the "unelected, non-resident, appointee" Emergency Financial Manager in what she called a hostile act unprecedented in US history. Longtime resident and ninety-nine-year-old activist Grace Lee Boggs (2013) added, "Detroit's financial bankruptcy didn't happen overnight—or by accident. Racism played a huge role."

This historical summary of Detroit begins with these topical vignettes because that is where many readers may connect with the troubles of Detroit. Indeed, the spectacle of Detroit's economic decline, including its many abandoned, crumbling buildings and high rates of poverty and crime, tends to consume the image of the city and its people. However, for the sake of truly understanding the challenges of food justice, a minor goal of this article is to dispel the historical amnesia concerning Detroit's decline.

Today, Detroit is still known by the monikers "motor city" or "motown." This is due to the vast expansion of Detroit's automobile and defense industries in the early twentieth century. During World War II, it formed part of the US "Arsenal of Democracy," producing vast amounts of military machinery (Sugrue 2005). A few decades prior, Detroit was starting to receive attention for job opportunities like Henry Ford's 1914 promise of five dollars per day for autoworkers. Northern cities such as Detroit gained a great deal of economic prestige, especially amongst European immigrants and African Americans in the US South. Due largely to migration from the South, Detroit witnessed a boost in the African American population from 5,741 (1910) to 40,838 (1920) to 120,066 (1930). Overall, the city's population doubled between 1910 and 1920, from 465,766 to 993,678, and then doubled again to reach almost two million at its peak in 1950 (Martin 1992; White 2011a). The en masse movement of African Americans northward, later called the Great Migration, had an enormous influence on the future of northern cities like Detroit.

Many African American migrants in the early twentieth century were influenced by both the push of southern oppression and the pull of northern promise. Migrants journeyed north in search of a better livelihood and relief from the economic, social, and political restrictions of the Jim Crow South. In the Reconstruction Era following legal emancipation from slavery, African American farmers overcame many barriers to obtain landownership and economic independence. Indeed, by 1910, African Americans had acquired fifteen million acres of land—a great feat considering the underdevelopment experienced under slavery and that, by that same year, nearly every southern state had succeeded in disenfranchising black males who had received the right to vote with the fifteenth amendment (C. Gilbert 1999). In addition, the white southern elite used coercive violence and the agro-economic systems of tenancy, sharecropping, and the crop lien to maintain dominance and keep African Americans in states of indebtedness and dependency to white planters. African American farmers also faced discrimination from the US Department of Agriculture (USDA) and white-owned banks (Green, Green, and Kleiner 2011). Racial oppression and economic depressions in the 1920s and 1930s pushed many African American farmers off the land and to seek employment in the urban industries of the South and the North (C. Gilbert 1999).

When northern industrial cities began hiring labor agents to attract skilled and unskilled workers, black southerners were particularly drawn to the dual promise of economic opportunity and social equality (Martin 1992, City of Opportunity section). However, upon arrival, they found that where Jim Crow de jure (law-based) segregation was absent, the de facto segregation of "separate but unequal" was the norm (Tyner 2007, 223). Carter G. Woodson, remarking on the mass movement of African Americans in the Great Migration, suggested that "the maltreatment of the Negro [would] be nationalized by the exodus" (Martin 1992, City of Opportunity section). Indeed, black southerners encountered a world that perpetuated racial inequality by barring African Americans from access to coveted industrial jobs. Even when industry was booming and hundreds of factory workers were being hired each day, many African Americans suffered from racial discrimination in employment (Sugrue 2005). Then, with the onset of economic restructuring, economic inequalities became even more pronounced.

In the 1940s, deindustrialization began to shrink factories and leave thousands of workers unemployed. The economic downturn contributed to an "uncertain postwar social order" that white elites negotiated by facilitating the highly racialized movements of people, known as suburbanization or "white flight" (Tyner 2007, 224). The decline of the industrial economy coincided with the redesign of the city and the construction of a highway system to allow middle- and upper-class access to the suburbs. The new highways carefully avoided middle- and upper-class neighborhoods in favor of devastating low-income black areas, such as when the Chrysler (originally Oakland-Hastings) Freeway blasted through the Paradise Valley and Black Bottom neighborhoods, which were the residential, commercial, and cultural centers of Black Detroit up until the 1950s. Large public housing schemes were developed (often late) for displaced residents, but "urban renewal" failed to revive economies or even improve living conditions. Accordingly, James Tyner (2007, 225) argued that urban renewal schemes emerged "not out of any genuine concern for the welfare of inner-city residents, but rather as a means of recapturing urban economic bases and tax bases." The highway and urban renewal projects may have been deemed "slum-razing" tools for removing "blight," but, in reality, they displaced thousands of people and destroyed the social fabric of many black communities (Sugrue 2005, 47-48).

Whites continued to maintain separate social and economic spheres and to isolate economic decline in many low-income and black neighborhoods through tactics such as discriminatory real estate practices (i.e., homeowners associations, zoning, and redlining), restricted access to loans and economic opportunity, and inadequate public transportation systems (McClintock 2011; Tyner 2007). Across the United States, "black ghettos" became defined by debilitating social circumstances: "Joblessness, welfare dependency, and single parenthood become the norm, and crime and disorder are inextricably woven into the fabric of daily life" (Massey and Denton 1993, 118). The intentional economic and social degradation of the inner city through "ghettoization" severely limited the self-determination and self-sufficiency of these communities and caused many economic institutions, including food retailers, to flee the city.

In 2010, Detroit was recognized as the most segregated city in the United States and continues to reflect the trend of "chocolate city and vanilla suburbs" popularized in Parliament's 1975 hit song, "Chocolate City," about Washington, DC (White 2010). These trends signal the failed project of integration, but, more importantly, they directly link to conditions known as "food deserts." According to the USDA (2009), food deserts are areas with "limited access to affordable and nutritious food" (1). A 2007 study by Mari Gallagher on food deserts in Detroit found roughly 550,000 residents—over half of the city's population—living in areas with high degrees of food imbalance. Gallagher refined the concept of food deserts by measuring food imbalance as "the distance to the closest grocer divided by the distance to the closest fringe food location." Furthermore, Gallagher found that food imbalance increased the rates of diet-related health problems and premature death in a given area (4-5). Detroit-based scholar Monica White (2010, 197) elaborated on the spatial significance of this study: "The places where healthy food is found tend to be financially inaccessible and . . . geographically out of reach for local residents, many of whom have limited access to reliable transportation." Essentially, the concept of food deserts demonstrates the spatial elements of food insecurity.

While this spatial analysis can be helpful, its emphasis on the built environment of a particular area can sometimes simultaneously work to gloss over the agency of local folks and ignore the larger structural issues that produced the food insecurity. Therefore, in this article, I will use the term *food insecurity* most frequently, due to its potentially more apt and less distracting description of the challenge faced by low-income families in parts of Detroit. Through taking a historical perspective, we can see that the structural inequities of systemic racism and concentrated poverty (i.e., "ghettoization") via real estate and planning practices, economic divestment, and inadequate public transportation contribute directly to food insecurity in Detroit.

Racial injustice and the economic development strategies led by white elites went hand-in-hand to deprive many black communities of access to economic, social, and political power. It is no mistake or coincidence that marginalized farming people, who arrived in northern cities after being refused equal citizenship and an equitable place in the southern agricultural economy, were ghettoized and forced to continue living as second-class citizens. Systemic racism and uneven development are the roots of Detroit's troubles. Therefore, any attempt to construct a more sustainable and just food system must reckon with this history.

Justice in the Food Movement

> For black farmers, it is not a matter of going back to the days of yesteryear, for how can a system based on slavery and sharecropping be considered idyllic? Instead it is a matter of continuously striving to achieve justice in the future.
> —John J. Green, Eleanor M. Green, and Anna M. Kleiner, "From the Past to the Present"

In the "food deserts" of Detroit and elsewhere, residents have long-standing traditions of using small available plots to grow food. However, only recently has it been termed *urban agriculture* and associated with the burgeoning food movement. Popular writers such as Michael Pollan (2008) and Barbara Kingsolver (2007) have articulated some of the main tenets of the food movement, including organic, local, and slow food. These values often take the form of participation in farm-to-table restaurants, farmers markets, community gardens, and community-supported agriculture, or CSAs. To a large degree, the food movement has been dominated by middle- to upper-class white/European American values and, oftentimes unknowingly, has silenced the histories of nonwhite ethnic groups in relation to food and agriculture, dominating the discussion about how to deal with the problems of hunger, diet-related disease, and the environmental pollution of industrial agriculture (Alkon and Agyeman 2011). This section will introduce the concept of food justice and the existing scholarship on food movements within communities of color and poor communities.

Food justice activism has emerged from communities of color suffering directly from marginalization in the food system and various diet-related diseases. Given the cultural diversity involved in food justice, the broad definition provided by veteran organization Just Food is most appropriate: "Food justice is communities exercising their right to grow, sell, and eat [food that is] fresh, nutritious, affordable, culturally appropriate, and grown locally with care for the well-being of the land, workers, and animals" (Alkon and Agyeman 2011, 5). Within this definition, one can find attributes of what Agyeman (2008, 752) calls "transformative sustainability or *just* sustainability," which is the idea that sustainability, with its conventional environmental focus, undergoes a paradigm shift to a more redistributive framework in which "justice and equity must move centre stage."

In the next section, I will further unpack the characteristics of the emerging food justice movement, including its critiques of the food movement and its roots in communities of color in the United States.

One of the foremost problems of the food movement is the great irony with which it claims progress toward a more sustainable food system, and yet declines to address issues of equity and justice for all people. Michael Pollan notably stated, "Not everyone can afford to eat high-quality food in America, and that is shameful: however, those of us who can, should." Guthman (2011, 276) criticizes the exclusivity of his statement by observing that "what at first appears to be a compassionate statement . . . assumes the persistence of inequality and, for that matter, ignores that the racialized land and labor relationships embedded in the U.S. food system continue to contribute to structural inequality." The larger point here is that, despite its good intentions, the food movement often lacks attention to issues of equity and justice, even when ostensibly attending to unequal access. Part of the problem lies in the exclusionary practices of the food movement, which appeals most strongly to the white, middle- to upper-class clientele that comprise its ranks.

While the food movement often focuses on a universal goal of "knowing where your food comes from," the disregard for historical differences in experience with agriculture endangers the food movement's ability to truly correct or improve upon the abuses of the past. It assumes that all peoples are willing and able to participate in alternative food practices, including paying higher prices for food. Indeed, Guthman (2008b, 394) argues that asking marginalized communities to "pay the full cost" of organic food, for example, means "asking people who might have historical connections to those who have more than paid the cost with their bodies and livelihoods in U.S. agricultural development—who in certain respects have themselves subsidized the production of cheap food—*to pay even more*" (my emphasis). What Guthman pinpoints here is the great privileged inattention with which the dominant food movement has regarded the histories of systemic and structural inequalities that have historically impeded working class and nonwhite groups of people from full participation in various aspects of US society. Even in attempts to be sympathetic or, more actively, "fix" communities suffering from food insecurity, food movement activists tend to overlook these stories and focus on the largely white and middle-class strategies for change outlined above.

In response to the dominant food movement narratives, groups such as the Growing Food and Justice for All Initiative (GFJI) have developed a focus on issues of racial inequality that stem from the relative absence of people of color in the food movement. For example, one GFJI member, Ben Yahola of the American Indian-based Mvskoke Food Sovereignty Initiative, describes the work of reclaiming food and cultural sovereignty (Morales 2011, 163). By tying food to the history of European colonization, he asserts an agrarian vision based on his own cultural heritage. In another case, Malik Yakini (2012a) of the Detroit Black Community Food Security Network (DBCFSN) described the dominance of whites within the food movement as "a disturbing trend rooted in the on-going legacy of white supremacy and privilege that characterizes American society." While American Indian experiences of inequality in the food system is certainly distinct from that of African Americans, the numerous examples of communities of color addressing both food *and* justice demonstrate the need for cultural and historical awareness in the food justice movement.

Finally, the food justice movement has demonstrated a clear need for marginalized communities to have control over their own food systems, not only for the sake of sovereignty but because a growing body of literature shows that contemporary food systems are both socially unjust *and* environmentally unsustainable (Green, Green, and Kleiner 2011). Julian Agyeman (2008, 752), who investigates the compatibility of environmental justice and sustainability traditions in what he calls "just sustainability," writes unequivocally that "human inequality is bad for environmental quality." Various examples show that the industrial agri-food systems that have privileged large-scale farms and driven many small-scale and nonwhite farmers off the land have also been environmentally unsustainable (Berry 1977; Magdoff, Foster, and Buttel 2000; Alkon and Agyeman 2011). Various ethnic groups, such as the Karuk people in what is now California, Asian immigrant farmers, and Latino immigrant farmworkers, have been displaced from traditional ethnic forms of agriculture and incorporated into food systems that foster food insecurity and unsustainable practices (Norgaard, Reed, and Van Horn 2011; Minkoff-Zern et al. 2011; S. Brown and Getz 2011). African American farmers, in particular, have lost control in the food system via land displacement and an astounding "98 percent loss of black farm operations between 1900 and 1997 compared with a nearly 66 percent loss among white operations" (Green, Green, and Kleiner 2011, 55). Clearly, the increased mechanization, industrialization, and consolidation of food systems prevent many communities from defining and creating food systems that meet their needs, especially low-income and nonwhite communities. The remainder of this article is devoted to how one organization, the Feedom Freedom Growers (FFG), cultivates just sustainability, or the intersection of justice and sustainability, in the local food system through a model of black cultural capital and grassroots development.

Black Cultural Capital and Community in the Feedom Freedom Growers

> Nobody wants to live through a depression, and it is unfair, or at least deeply ironic, that black people in Detroit are being forced to undertake an experiment in utopian post-urbanism that appears to be uncomfortably similar to the sharecropping past their parents and grandparents sought to escape. There is no moral reason why they should do and be better than the rest of us—but there is a practical one. They have to.
> —Rebecca Solnit, "Detroit Arcadia"

As this article has shown, the decline of industrial Detroit and enduring racial inequality devastated African American communities socially, economically, and environmentally. Therefore, in grassroots responses that seek popular participation in social change, community building is a key component. In an example specific to postindustrial contexts, Helen Matthews Lewis (2009) articulated community building as the defining feature of grassroots or participatory development in post-mining industry towns of Appalachia. In her "Twelve Step Program for Recovering from Industrial Recruitment," Lewis begins with "1. Understand your history—share memories" and "2. Mobilize/organize/revive a sense of community" (74). Lewis demonstrates how a sense of community, as generated through storytelling and recognizing the value of traditional methods of "raising and preserving food and home remedies," is vital to grassroots development (81).

Similarly, in response to the question of how to redevelop Detroit following the decline of the automobile industry and the reality of increasing "social alienation, violence, and insecurity within black communities" in the 1980s and 1990s, the activists James and Grace

Lee Boggs recognized the need for community building (Ward 2011, 318). Through a variety of projects and activities, such as "community gardens, . . . recycling projects, . . . neighborhood responsibility councils, repair shops, skills banks, panels to resolve disputes between neighbors, and community bakeries," they hoped communities would develop "collective self-reliance through which citizens could rely on themselves—and not city (or state or national) government—to revitalize Detroit and other cities" (319). Likewise, the Feedom Freedom Growers (FFG) has committed to the long-term process of community building by developing personal relationships with neighbors, bonding over common experiences and cultural backgrounds, and collectively proposing alternatives in the pursuit of food justice.

The FFG is a small organization of mostly African Americans on the east side of Detroit dedicated to fostering food justice. The organization operates programs in art, education, growing food for the purpose of "cultivating self-reliance that sustains the life of our developing communities" (Feedom Freedom Growers 2012). Cofounders Myrtle Thompson and Wayne Curtis began in 2008 with a small vegetable garden beside their home. In the years that followed, the organization grew to involve many of their children—Kezia, Tyrone, Monique, Travis, and Shereece—all of whom were in their early twenties to early thirties. In addition to family members, the FFG has relied on like-minded people who work or volunteer for the organization for varying periods of time. The organization has steadily developed youth programs for the many unexpected children who regularly visit the garden and attend community programs such as block parties and roundtable discussions (see appendix A). As a predominantly black organization serving a predominantly black neighborhood, the FFG has built its programs, philosophies, and strategies for food justice using elements of black culture and history.

In order to facilitate community building, the FFG has used black cultural capital to help create bonds and guide the content and form of their activism. The term *cultural capital* describes how shared identities, consciousness, and behaviors function for instrumental and expressive purposes. For example, an instrumental purpose might support the social and economic development of a community, whereas an expressive purpose might demonstrate in-group affiliation (Carter 2003). Bettye Collier-Thomas (2004) provides an example of how black women used various fundraising skills and techniques (such as bake sales, rummage sales, and dinners), imbued with a sense of group consciousness and collective identity, as cultural capital to support educational and charitable institutions in the black community. While food preparation skills are only a minor point in Collier-Thomas's analysis, I want to point out the integral nature of agricultural and food preparation practices, or agri-food practices, to the identity and survival of a culture. For African Americans, agri-food practices began on the African continent (e.g., rice farming on West African coast) and have evolved through different experiences with land, agriculture, and food in the United States (Carney 2001).

The revolutionary nature of growing food in historically oppressed areas of Detroit rests on the FFG's understanding of black cultural capital and grassroots development as integral parts of their food justice activism. As articulated in their slogan "grow a garden, grow a community," FFG members talked frequently about the need to involve community members in their grassroots efforts. Why? Tyrone suggested succinctly that "Baba [Wayne] always says that revolution is impossible without the community. . . . And that's one thing that Huey [Newton] taught too: you can't survive without the support of your community." This response captured a few of the main characteristics of FFG's strategy for social change: a dedication to community building and the history of the black freedom movement. Wayne's experiences as a member of the Black Panther Party (BPP) in Detroit during the 1970s served as a major inspiration for the organization.

When Huey P. Newton and Bobby Seale founded the BPP in Oakland in 1966, they aimed to address "the historical unwillingness of the U.S. government to provide viable welfare services to unemployed African Americans and other minorities living in inner cities" (Heynen 2009, 410). The BPP used a combination of grassroots organizing and mutual aid "survival programs" to pool resources from the community in order to help satisfy immediate needs in health care, education, and food. The BPP responded to their observation that many children went to school hungry by establishing the Free Breakfast for Children Program, which fed thousands of children each day before school (Heynen 2009). The community building tactics used by the BPP demonstrate how black radical organizations have, for generations, fought against inequality in the food system by building spaces of collective self-reliance.

In acknowledging that black people in the United States have "never had the support of institutions [run by the nation-state]," Wayne emphasized the BPP's relevance in black history: "We [black Americans] have always had to build the space . . . always had to build this entity in which we could determine our destiny and resolve our problems, and create the structures that *we* would sustain, to take care of and perform certain duties for us in certain areas: education, housing, medical . . . because we were lacking that connection with the so-called institutions under capitalism. So we had to do this ourselves." Wayne's description of the insights he gained in the BPP regarding autonomous spaces feed directly into the goals of the FFG to reclaim land for urban agriculture and use community building as the framework for grassroots development (Tyner 2006). In contrast with the "industrial recruitment model" discussed by Lewis or a model overly reliant on government services, the BPP built parallel institutions to satisfy community needs. Thus, Wayne's discussion of self-reliance to meet community needs resonates strongly with the radical politics of the BPP.

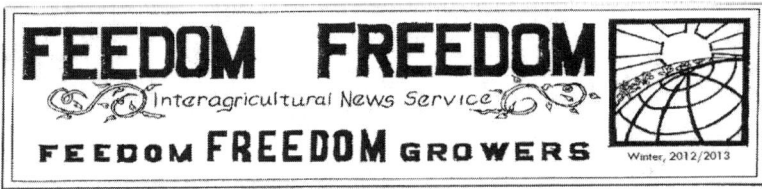

Another prominent reference to the BPP appeared in the FFG's newsletter publication, entitled "Feedom Freedom: The Interagricultural News Service" (see illustration above). As a Black Panther, Wayne often worked as a salesman for the BPP's newspaper called the *Intercommunal News Service* in order to raise money for projects in his Detroit chapter and the developing base in Oakland, California. The idea of intercommunalism promoted self-determination in local communities while linking the efforts to the larger struggle for black communities in the United States and around the world. The news service served as a communication tool between BPP chapters across the country and also to keep BPP members informed about revolutionary movements throughout the African Diaspora and Third World, like Samora Machel's in Mozambique, which Wayne noted as an important influence. Similarly, the FFG newsletter has helped inform others about their work and link them to other groups fighting for food justice in Detroit and elsewhere.

Finally, a reference to the BPP appeared in a youth's creative work entitled, "A Food Justice Poem," published in the Winter 2012/2013 newsletter:

Creepy, crawly, flying insects
Eww . . .
Compost, touching it
Gross . . .
Justice over food??
Whatever . . .

Fighting for what's right
Hoping for a new Wall Street
The government may ignore our cries
But like the Black Panthers,
We will NOT be beat by our own fight!

Then came Us kids
Who believed we could change the world
We closed our old ways and ideas
And we were opened to a new life
We knew it didn't come without a price!

Using experiences with the FFG, the young person drew a comparison between the activism of the BPP and the FFG. Specifically, the description of having to "[close] our old ways and ideas" resonates with how Wayne described "working through contradictions" in the BPP—making personal and collective changes in ideas and behaviors when necessary to address community needs. The poem provides evidence of how the content and form of activism by the BPP is passed down to the FFG's youth participants in the form of black cultural capital. Their example and common black identity serve as encouragement for the FFG's youth participants to also struggle dialectically for justice.

In contrast to the inspiration drawn from the black cultural capital of the BPP, the collective memory of slavery poses the challenge of reframing agriculture as a potential source of power. Monique, discussing her frustrations with getting people involved with the FFG, said, "There are a lot of people who don't wanna work in the garden because they feel like slaves working in the field." Yakini of the DBCFSN described the problem in a similar way: "Part of the challenge we have with organizing African Americans for this work is that many of our people associate this work with enriching somebody else, associate it with slavery or sharecropping, both of which enriched whites through our labor. And part of what we're doing is reframing agriculture for African Americans, so that we can again see it as an act of self-determination and self-empowerment." (Democracy Now! 2010) Indeed, the stigma attached to agriculture for some in the black community is a strong indication of an enduring association between agriculture and the conditions of slavery and of the ongoing challenges facing small-scale and minority farmers. However, evidence of a positive reframing of agriculture is evident in Myrtle's declaration that the example set by the DBCFSN as a well-organized and "unapologetically black" organization helped her to attach a positive racial sentiment to food justice activism.

Another important part of the FFG's reframing strategy was establishing connections with Detroiters who have southern roots. Although geographically outside of the US South, the FFG can maintain cultural connections with the South through food. Myrtle related how many of the people who have "stopped [by]" or who "appreciate the food that we raise here are from the South." She pointed out that a nearby pastor "from the South" was one of their biggest supporters and had helped them till the soil during the first growing season because he had "always grown his own food." Not only that, he also had chickens, which Myrtle assured me was not rare: "People have had chickens forever in Detroit. Chickens don't make noise. They neighbors know but they don't bother anybody." She also described an "elderly, beautiful little lady" who, although she did not get out of the house much anymore, walked down the street on a walking stick to see the garden and share stories about how she used to grow "her food by the moon." This encounter, in particular, Myrtle described with a sense of utter appreciation and love: "For her to come down here, it was just like, it was too much . . . little things like that." Overall, Myrtle drew connections between the current urban agriculture movement, a longer history of Detroiters (including her grandparents) growing food in the city, and an even longer heritage of agriculture rooted in southern African American communities and, even, African communities. The connections seemed to give her a sense of pride and cultural continuity: encouraging her not to frame agriculture as a shameful practice despite its association with the oppressive and inhumane conditions of chattel slavery and sharecropping systems.

I also found that the FFG framed agriculture in a longer historical view reaching back to their African ancestors and to food issues on the continent of Africa. For example, at the block party event in July, they provided pamphlets about food and politics, including a short essay entitled "African State of Mind," by James Sheely, which critiqued the lack of recognition for African contributions to agriculture: "It's hard to imagine how someone could talk about agriculture and fail to bring up Africa, especially when addressing a room full of African descendants." The article went on to describe the birth of agriculture in Kush (modern-day Ethiopia) and how agriculture sustained the development of culture in areas of "mathematics, language, music . . . government, medicine, religion." By providing an alternative narrative about the history of agriculture and development, the FFG challenges the dominance of the white agrarian story in the US food movement.

Throughout the FFG's community building, the organization focuses on cultivating relationships and avoiding top-down instructions about food choices. When I asked Kezia about their strategies for outreach, she replied that she did not think of it as outreach but as community building. She related how when they passed out flyers or talked to people about food and health, they were not seeking to impose a new diet on people. Rather, Kezia asserted how face-to-face dialogue and long-term commitment allowed people to trust the organization: "People know that they're not just gonna up and disappear. Mama Myrtle and Baba Wayne, they live in the community, they love this community, they a part of this community, so it's not just somebody trying to come in and exploit me or my family or my community. . . . How do you expect them to get onboard with you if you're not willing to support them and listen to what they have to say?" Kezia also stressed the importance of allowing people to "formulate their own questions and their own thoughts about something versus saying, 'this is a food desert. You should be pissed,' [without addressing the basic questions], like, why don't we have any food? What is really going on in this community? . . . The food that we do have access to, why is it not good?" As a grassroots organization whose members also live in food desert conditions, the FFG has developed grassroots participation by carefully dialoguing with community members in order to build relationships and collectively name the barriers to food justice.

One evening while several FFG members and I were playing Apples to Apples, a card game based on making humorous connections between words, an association was proposed between the words *fast food* and *fake*. Myrtle interjected by reminding us that fast food often seemed like the only option for many people and that we shouldn't disparage those food choices. This topic reemerged a few weeks later at a roundtable discussion that the older youth facilitated on the topic of food justice. Since the event had drawn neighborhood youth, parents, and other urban growers and supporters in

Detroit, the discussion presented a good opportunity to recognize the multiple meanings of food justice. Interestingly, the group was clearly supportive of an urban grower who disliked the way people were criticized or insulted for certain food choices, especially fast food choices, when there were economic reasons or even sentimental reasons behind the choice. Therefore, instead of emphasizing a sense of moral superiority over people who choose fast foods, the FFG encourages an atmosphere accepting of all food choices while attempting to create new, healthier attachments to foods by teaching people how to grow, cook, and introduce new foods into their diet.

This perspective on fast food reflects essential elements of dialogue in that, as Paolo Freire (1970, 90) suggests, "Dialogue cannot exist without humility. . . . How can I dialogue if I consider myself a member of the in-group of 'pure' men, the owners of truth and knowledge, for whom all non-members are 'these people' or 'the great unwashed?'" Whereas the dominant food movement tends to valorize local, organic food production over industrial food production without considering issues of equity, the FFG acknowledges the limited food choices of Detroiters who live in food deserts and enacts a more grassroots approach to identifying and responding to food needs.

Overall, the use of black cultural capital throughout the various components of grassroots development formed a powerful framework for engaging and building community. The FFG's food justice activism rejected the unrelenting attention to expensive local and organic food and focused on encouraging the cultural attachments that community members make with specific foods. The FFG used black cultural capital to connect with everyone from elderly black southerners to Detroit-born youth on the importance of food justice and self-reliance in gardening and cooking.

A Vision of Just Sustainability in Detroit

> The revolution to be made in the United States will be the first revolution in history to require the masses to make material sacrifices rather than acquire more material things. We must give up many of the things which this country has enjoyed at the expense of damning over one-third of the world into a state of underdevelopment, ignorance, disease, and early death.
>
> —James and Grace Lee Boggs, *Revolution and Evolution in the Twentieth Century*

As demonstrated in the previous section, the FFG manifests some of the most important attributes of food justice activism in the African American community: the use of black cultural capital to root themselves within the predominantly African American community and a grassroots development style that prioritizes popular participation and community relationships. This last section will delve further into the idea of grassroots development by looking at the concept of just sustainability in contrast to conventional economic development.

The vision of grassroots development in the Detroit urban agriculture movement begins with reclaiming land that has been abandoned by private owners and city officials. Like the lyrics of Detroit rapper Danny Brown's 2012 song "Fields," the landscape of Detroit is replete with the recurrent images of "house, field, field / field, field, house / abandoned house, field, field." According to the Detroit Food Policy Council (2012), there are 106,000 vacant lots in the city, 60 percent of which are owned by the city government. Travis described the City of Detroit's lack of responsibility in taking care of the vacant lots it owns and the unfairness of its practices regarding land: The city "ain't even cutting the grass on this land they talking about people can't get or grow some food on or play a game of football on without the police pulling up telling people they can't play. . . . What they trying to do with the land is not benefitting the people that live on the land and that don't make no sense to me." Despite the city's unfair practices, people had been reclaiming vacant land for urban agriculture for decades. Taking matters into their own hands, Detroiters have bypassed the city to make use of the land for personal and communal benefit.

The city government and prospective developers, however, often do not recognize urban gardens as legitimate contributions to the city and its communities. Kezia related the uncritical process of the city government labeling lots as vacant: "As far as the city is concerned, without looking at this [pointing to the FFG garden], this is a vacant lot in the city. And so on paper, people that are outside the city read that there are 300 or however many vacant lots. It's not really a true statement, but there's no one to say different. They don't have any other voice there to say, 'no'." Whereas individual communities and families had already made joint decisions to use the land for self-help purposes, the city government then had the potential to (and often did) take back land in accordance with obsolete food and land-use policies. This type of conflict has emerged in many cities across the country where urban agriculture is on the rise (Voigt 2011).

A major conflict over food and land-use policy soon emerged over the Hantz Farm/Woodlands proposal to purchase two thousand city-owned lots (at $300 each) in order to eventually create a ten-thousand-acre "farm" (see appendix B). Despite how the owner of the project, John Hantz, masqueraded the proposal in progressive urban agriculture terminology, the urban agriculture community soon recognized his real intentions to raise property values by creating "land scarcity," which some compared to "a classic land grab—with all its disastrous consequences" (Holt-Giménez 2012). In opposition to the top-down style of development employed by Hantz, members of the Detroit Food Policy Council (DFPC) and DBCFSN created a counterproposal for a community land trust, which was designed to "ensure community benefits and keep land in the hands of the people who have been here for generations." Their argument is based on the "the grounds that there exist no clear processes for buying land and that this transaction only exacerbates the land inequality status quo amongst the haves and have-nots" (Thompson 2012). The community land trust ultimately presented a larger vision of community landholding as part of a grassroots development approach (see appendix C).

Part of the problem existed in how, according to Myrtle, a local organization called the Lower Eastside Action Plan (LEAP) acted as a "gatekeeper" for Hantz to suggest that his organization had "community buy-in." Meanwhile, Hantz had actually avoided the DFPC and other urban agriculture organizations, including the FFG, throughout the planning process (Holt-Giménez 2012). Wayne reinforced this idea by asserting that the urban agriculture community was not heard and contrasting the two models: "To me, they don't care anything about our response. . . . They're just steady going forward to get the land. They don't care what we say, what we want . . . [but] the community land trust says that we want to use the land for our benefit." For Wayne, the community land trust is only part of a larger vision for a grassroots approach to just sustainability:

> Legally we have to have access to the land—pure and simple—and that's what the fight is over. Land is private property to make money for the economy and that's what they talk about. One of the mayoral candidates supports Hantz and he said it's good for the economy, for the GDP (Gross Domestic Product). Hantz is good for that. But the things we want to do is not good for the GDP: we're talking about riding bikes . . . riding bikes to the store to

buy a tomato that was grown in the neighborhood. That's not doing much for the GDP. I didn't buy gas. The car's not gonna break down. I'm not contributing to the global agricultural system . . . where that money goes—I'm studying that—how that money circulates within Wall St. We're not good for that. . . . That's what the contradiction is. So, automatically, without even understanding who we are, what we represent, without even understanding the degrading of human beings and non-human beings, they're against [us]. They have no consciousness of what bio-centrism is: a culture that considers *all life* instead of being centered on the survival of human beings.

Wayne's analysis of the Hantz proposal and the goals of the FFG demonstrates the vast differences in how they envision the (re)development of Detroit. I share this extended quote not only because of how Wayne seamlessly links social, economic, and environmental concerns into a single vision of change but also for how the complexity of such issues indicates the need for a slower process and a fundamentally different vision of development.

The FFG's vision of a slower process of development demonstrates a commitment to more fundamental changes and a long-term relationship with the community. Myrtle specifically critiqued the pace with which the Hantz proposal was pushed through: "It didn't have to be a rushed job. It wasn't necessary. They [the city government] could've charged and made so much more for that land. They could've made him [Hantz] come out with a really detailed plan." But what does the FFG offer as the alternative? "We gotta much slower process . . . more tedious but more sustainable overall. It's more equitable and fair for everyone . . . if you really wanna shift it [the status quo], you gotta be willing to change some things." The slower pace seemingly allows for more consideration of different opinions and a more equitable process.

The FFG also demonstrates the interconnectedness of various movements for just sustainability. The work of the FFG also depends on the work of organizations like Fender Bender, "a women, transgender, and queer justice-based bike shop and mechanic training experience," with which Kezia is an active participant (Fender Bender Detroit). Fender Bender's work may appear unrelated to the FFG's, but these organizations complement each other, from an ecofeminist perspective, by connecting "the oppression and pollution of the earth with their own oppression and view[ing] the earth as an ally," and by addressing just sustainability in key aspects of community livelihood (food and transportation, respectively) (White 2011b, 25). But can these movements accumulate enough power to challenge the dominant systems? If so, how?

Some of the FFG described the challenge of developing self-reliance while fulfilling daily needs or, as Tyrone described it, some people staying "on the plantation while some dig a hole to help get out." Myrtle elaborated further about this array of problems for activists:

> Ok, we got these [activist] organizations but we also have to keep ourselves afloat because 9 times out of 10 these non-profit organizations are not able to sustain what I'm doing: my lifestyle, my income, my bills, my gas, my lights, my rent. But it's the work that keeps me going . . . [but] there might be two different things going on . . . [until] my life and my work are synched up. . . . There are lots of folks that would like to just come out here and build with us, but "look, I gotta go do dah-dah-dah." And until we can figure out a way to unplug ourselves from Detroit Edison, the gas company, the rent mortgages, and stuff like that, and spend our time building, then that's what we have to deal with. And that's where I'm thinking a lot of the time: how do I unplug and get with the alternatives so that the real-life can happen?

Like other members of the FFG, Myrtle described a desire for self-reliance in making a living for herself and her family. Similar to how Wayne diminished the importance of GDP in measuring economic stability, Travis offered another vision of how urban agriculture produces self-reliance and wealth: "I'm putting all this life back in the earth and when it comes out the ground I get to harvest all this fresh food that I can't get from the store because even the fruits and the vegetables at the stores doesn't have all the nutrients as when I go outside and get the food from the side of my house." Travis continued by saying that the work of urban agriculture went "deeper than dollar signs," and explained, "just 'cause I'm not getting paid for it doesn't mean I'm not getting rich from it." Therefore, the vision of food sovereignty involves redefining economics not only in terms of keeping money in the local area but also in terms of the metrics used to calculate economic stability. By gradually "unplugging" from conventional economic development, turning to self-reliant alternatives, and consolidating wealth in forms such as nutrition and health, the FFG offers a nuanced understanding of changing the food system to generate more just sustainability.

Overall, we begin to see a vision of food justice that incorporates several different elements of just sustainability. First, the FFG's food justice activism has strong roots in the justice-oriented politics of black radical organizations like the BPP and their Free Breakfast for Children Program. Second, the FFG showed commitment to bottom-up grassroots development by not making value judgments on food choices, centering the work of community building, and by engaging people in culturally relevant ways. Third, the reclaiming of vacant land for urban agriculture by historically oppressed people signals a movement toward a more sustainable and just food system. And, fourth, measuring the success of food justice activism not only by the pounds of fresh, nutrient-dense foods grown but by the ability to "unplug" from conventional economic development indicates a deep commitment to both justice and sustainability.

Appendix A

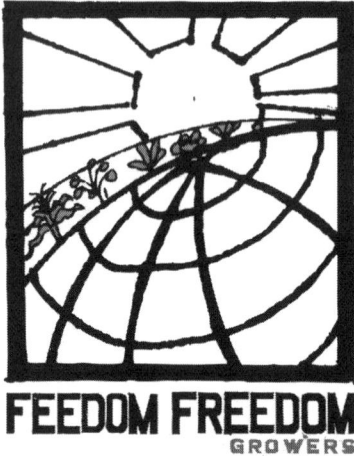

Community Roundtable Discussion

The revitalization of Detroit
through the speeches of
Dr. Martin Luther King, Jr.

Saturday, January 15th
11am-1pm

Hope Community Church
14456 E Jefferson

Feedom Freedom hosted its first roundtable discussion in October to open conversation around how we can continue to rebuild our communities through its best resource - the people. We intend to build on that conversation at this follow-up roundtable discussion, with a focus on how to rebuild Detroit through a selection of Martin Luther King, Jr.'s speeches.

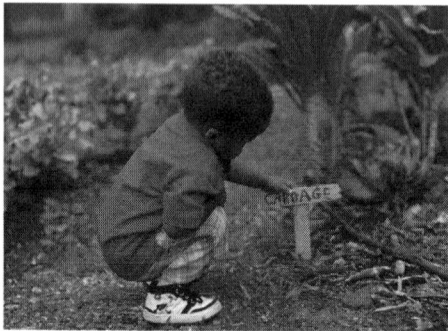

Appendix B

BLOCK BY BLOCK BY BLOCK BY BLOCK BY BLOCK BY BLOCK BY BLOCK BY BLOCK BY BLOCK BY BLOCK BY BLOCK

Detroit Land Grab!

This proposed sale of public land to Hantz Woodlands would sell over 1900 lots of vacant land for $300 a lot without any accountability around future development. There is concern that this sale, if approved, could set a precedent for future large-scale land sales.

It is reported that Hantz Woodlands is also attempting to purchase about 128 lots from the Michigan Land Bank Authority, lots located in this same footprint.

Please call City Council and, if possible, **attend the Council meeting on Tuesday, Nov 20th at 10 AM at Coleman A. Young Municipal Center** and participate in Public Comment.

#HANTZOFF
#LANDGRAB
#DETROITFUTURE

Stared lots are included in the proposed sale

$300! $300! $300! $300! $300! $300! $300!

MACK AVE

VAN DYKE ST

ST JEAN

JEFFERSON AVE

$300! $300! $300! $300! $300! $300! $300! $300!

WE NEED A PUBLIC HEARING ON THIS SALE!
WE NEED TO KNOW WHAT IS GOING TO BE DONE WITH THIS LAND!
WE NEED A CITY LAND BUYING PROCESS THAT IS FAIR AND JUST!

BLOCK BY BLOCK BY BLOCK BY BLOCK BY BLOCK BY BLOCK BY BLOCK BY BLOCK BY BLOCK BY BLOCK BY BLOCK

'JUST FEED DETROIT' HOTLINE
313.355.3121

Please Call for regular Updates and to 'share your story'

$300! $300! $300! $300! $300! $300! $300!

Blocks add up to Acres!

The number of acres about to be sold to **ONE MAN?**
180 ACRES!
One Hundred and Eighty Acres
= more than **1800 Lots!**

That's Lots of LAND!
Were YOU aware of this deal? Many are not!

Block this injustice with community action!
Resist this land grab right from under our noses!

Are you concerned about this preferential treatment?
Are you concerned that some are able to bypass the system?
Are you concerned what will be DONE with this land?

Did you know that, **as a resident, you have the right to purchase the land adjacent (next to) your home if its vacant?**

Did you know that making a call to City Council is one way to make your concerns known about YOUR RIGHTS as a citizen and community member? **CALL TODAY!**

Call Detroit City Council Members Today!

CHARLES PUGH
313.224.4510
CouncilPresidentPugh@detroitmi.gov

GARY BROWN
(313) 224-2450
councilmemberbrown@detroitmi.gov

SAUNTEEL JENKINS
(313) 224-4248
councilmemberjenkins@detroitmi.gov

KENNETH V. COCKREL, JR
(313) 224-4505
Kenneth.Cockrel@detroitmi.gov

BRENDA JONES
(313) 224-1245
bjones_mb@detroitmi.gov

ANDRÉ L. SPIVEY
(313) 224-4841
CouncilmanSpivey@detroitmi.gov

JAMES TATE
(313) 224-1027
councilmembertate@detroitmi.gov

KWAME KENYATTA
(313) 224-1198
K-Kenyatta_MB@detroitmi.gov

JOANN WATSON
(313) 224-4535
WatsonJ@detroitmi.gov

$300! $300! $300! $300! $300! $300!

BLOCK BY BLOCK BY BLOCK BY BLOCK BY BLOCK BY BLOCK BY BLOCK BY BLOCK BY BLOCK BY BLOCK BY BLOCK

Appendix C

COMMUNITY! LAND! TRUST!

John Hantz is attempting to purchase 1900 lots (180 Acres) of public land in your neighborhood for use as an industrial tree farm - HANTZ WOODLANDS.

The alternative to Hantz Woodlands? Set up a Community Land Trust (CLT) to ensure community benefits and keep land in the hands of the people who have lived here for generations. "CLT's balance the needs of individuals to access land and maintain security of tenure with a community's need to maintain affordability, economic diversity and local access to essential services."

Main issues with this ever-changing deal between Hantz Woodlands and The City of Detroit

1 Hantz is purchasing land for $300 per lot. THIS LAND, the community's land, which is right next to the Riverfront on an international border, in close proximity to Downtown, Belle Isle and City Airport, is of great value and importance, especially to the people who currently live there.

2 Sets a precedent for future land sales. This is the biggest land sale in Detroit history!! Hantz's original plan was 2,000 acres – will he stop at 180 acres?

3 Priority given to corporations over community. Citizens meet resistance from city when buying lots, while Hantz is dangerously close to buying up 1900 lots in one deal.

4 No commitment to community benefits for those most impacted. Hantz has no obligation to the long-term wellbeing of the community, this generation or the next.

5 Negative health effects. Exposure to pesticides can cause cancer, birth defects, and increase asthma symptoms!! Also environmental risks.

6 Lack of awareness. The community has intentionally been kept in the dark. This plan has been in the works for 3 years yet most residents are unaware. Now you know, don't be silent!

7 Continues tradition of displacement and disenfranchisement!! At this point homeowners are not being directly forced out, but there are concerns that this could be a long-term displacement strategy. Think South Jefferson.

PLEASE JOIN US TO SUPPORT A COMMUNITY LAND TRUST

MONDAY DECEMBER 10TH PUBLIC HEARING

East Lake Baptist Church (12400 E. Jefferson at Conner)

Rally at **5pm** Hearing at **6pm**

SAY NO TO HANTZ WOODLANDS!

SAY YES TO COMMUNITY LAND TRUST!

Works Cited

Agyeman, Julian. 2008. "Toward a Just Sustainability." *Continuum: Journal of Media & Cultural Studies* 22 (6): 751-56.

Agyeman, Julian, Robert D. Bullard, and Bob Evans. 2002. "Exploring the Nexus: Bringing Together Sustainability, Environmental Justice and Equity." *Space and Polity* 6 (1): 77-90.

Alkon, Alison Hope. 2012. *Black, White, and Green: Farmers Markets, Race, and the Green Economy*. Athens, GA: University of Georgia Press.

Alkon, Alison Hope, and Julian Agyeman, 2011. "Introduction: The Food Movement as Polyculture." In *Cultivating Food Justice: Race, Class, and Sustainability*, edited by Alison Hope Alkon and Julian Agyeman, 1-20. Cambridge, MA: MIT Press.

Berry, Wendell. 1977. *The Unsettling of America: Culture & Agriculture*. San Francisco: Sierra Club Books.

Boggs, Grace Lee. 2011. *The Next American Revolution: Sustainable Activism for the 21st Century*. Berkeley: University of California Press.

————. 2013. "Detroit's Bankruptcy and Resilience." *Michigan Citizen*, August 1. http://michigancitizen.com/detroits-bankruptcy-and-resilience.

Boggs, James, and Grace Lee Boggs. (1974) 2008. *Revolution and Evolution in the Twentieth Century*. 2nd ed. New York: Monthly Review.

Bowers, Chet A. 2001. *Educating for Eco-Justice and Community*. Athens: University of Georgia Press.

Brown, Danny. 2012. "Fields." On *XXX*. Brooklyn, NY: Fool's Gold Records, compact disc.

Brown, Elaine. 2007. "The Significance of the Newspaper of the Black Panther Party." In *The Black Panther: Intercommunal News Service 1967-1980*, edited by David Hilliard, ix-xi. New York: Atria Books.

Brown, Sandy, and Christy Getz. 2011. "Farmworker Food Insecurity and the Production of Hunger in California." In *Cultivating Food Justice: Race, Class, and Sustainability*, edited by Alison Hope Alkon and Julian Agyeman, 121-46. Cambridge, MA: MIT Press.

Carney, Judith. 2001. Black Rice: *The African Origins of Rice Cultivation in the Americas*. Cambridge: Harvard University Press.

Carter, Prudence. 2003. "'Black' Cultural Capital, Status Positioning, and Schooling Conflicts for Low-Income African American Youth." *Social Problems* 50 (1): 136-55.

Collier-Thomas, Bettye. 2004. "'Sister Laborers': African American Women, Cultural Capital, and Educational Philanthropy, 1865-1970." In *Cultural Capital and Black Education*, edited by V. P. Franklin and Carter Julian Savage, 97-115. Greenwich, CT: Information Age Publishing.

Democracy Now! 2010. "Detroit Urban Agriculture Movement Looks to Reclaim Motor City." Democracy Now! Video, June 24, video. http://www.democracynow.org/2010/6/24/detroit_urban_agriculture_movement_looks_to.

Detroit Food Policy Council. 2012. "Public Land Sale Process in Detroit: A Community Perspective." http://detroitfoodpolicycouncil.net/Reports.html.

Dolan, Matthew. 2012. "New Detroit Farm Plan Taking Root." *Wall Street Journal*, July 6. http://online.wsj.com/news/articles/SB10001424052702304898704577479090390757800.

Feedom Freedom Growers. 2012. Feedom Freedom Interagricultural News Service, Winter.

Fender Bender Detroit's Facebook page. 2013. Accessed January 24. https://www.facebook.com/FenderBenderCollective.

Freire, Paulo. 1970. *Pedagogy of the Oppressed.* New York: Continuum International Publishing Group.

Gallagher, Mari. 2007. "Examining the Impacts of Food Deserts on the Public Health in Detroit." Chicago: Mari Gallagher Research and Consulting Group, Chicago. http://www.marigallagher.com/projecs/2/.

Gilbert, Charlene. 1999. *Homecoming: Sometimes I am Haunted by Memories of Red Dirt and Clay.* San Francisco: California Newsreel. DVD.

Gilbert, Jess, Gwen Sharp, and M. Sindy Felin. 2002. "The Loss and Persistence of Black-Owned Farms and Farmland: A Review of the Research Literature and its Implications." *Southern Rural Sociology* 18 (2): 1-30.

Green, John J., Eleanor M. Green, and Anna M. Kleiner. 2011. "From the Past to the Present: Agricultural Development and Black Farmers in the American South." In *Cultivating Food Justice: Race, Class, and Sustainability*, edited by Alison Hope Alkon and Julian Agyeman, 47-64. Cambridge, MA: MIT Press.

Guthman, Julie. 2008a. "Bringing Good Food to Others: Investigating the Subjects of Alternative Food Practice." *Cultural Geographies* 15:431-47.

———. 2008b. "'If They Only Knew': Color Blindness and Universalism in California Alternative Food Institutions." *Professional Geographer* 60 (3): 387-97.

_____. 2011. "'If They Only Knew': The Unbearable Whiteness of Alternative Food." In *Cultivating Food Justice: Race, Class, and Sustainability*, edited by Alison Hope Alkon and Julian Agyeman, 263-81. Cambridge, MA: MIT Press.

Heynen, Nik. 2009. "Bending the Bars of Empire from Every Ghetto for Survival: The Black Panther Party's Radical Antihunger Politics of Social Reproduction and Scale." *Annals of the Association of American Geographers* 99 (2): 406-22.

Holt-Giménez, Eric. 2011. "Food Security, Food Justice, or Food Sovereignty?: Crises, Food Movements, and Regime Change." In *Cultivating Food Justice: Race, Class, and Sustainability*, edited by Alison Hope Alkon and Julian Agyeman, 309-30. Cambridge, MA: MIT Press.

_____. 2012. "Detroit: A Tale of Two . . . Farms?" *Huffington Post*, July 10. http://www.huffingtonpost.com/eric-holt-gimenez/a-tale-of-two-farms_b_1660019.html.

Holt-Giménez, Eric, and Yi Wang. 2011. "Reform or Transformation?: The Pivotal Role of Food Justice in the U.S. Food Movement." *Race/Ethnicity: Multidisciplinary Global Contexts* 5 (1): 83-102.

Isidore, Chris. 2013. "Detroit Files for Bankruptcy." CNN, July 18th. http://money.cnn.com/2013/07/18/news/economy/detroit-bankruptcy/index.html.

Kingsolver, Barbara, with Steven L. Hopp and Camille Kingsolver. 2007. *Animal, Vegetable, Miracle: A Year of Food Life*. New York: Harper Collins.

Lewis, Helen Matthew. 2009. "Rebuilding Communities: A Twelve-Step Recovery Program." In *Participatory Development in Appalachia: Cultural Identity, Community, and*

Sustainability, edited by Susan E. Keefe, 67-88. Knoxville: University of Tennessee Press.

Magdoff, Fred, John Bellamy Foster, and Frederick H. Buttel, eds. 2000. *Hungry for Profit: The Agribusiness Threat to Farmers, Food, and the Environment*. New York: Monthly Review Press.

Massey, Douglas S., and Nancy A. Denton. 1993. *American Apartheid: Segregation and the Making of the Underclass*. Cambridge, MA: Harvard University Press.

Martin, Elizabeth Anne. 1992. "Detroit and the Great Migration 1916-1929." *Bentley Historical Library*. http://bentley.umich. edu/research/publications/migration/index.php.

Maynard, Melissa. 2013. "Detroit's Bankruptcy Complicates Relationship with Michigan State Government." *Huffington Post*, July 31. http://www.huffingtonpost.com/2013/07/31/ detroit-bankruptcy-michigan-government-state-relationship_n_3682617.html.

McClintock, Nathan. 2011. "From Industrial Garden to Food Desert: Demarcated Devaluation in the Flatlands of Oakland, California." In *Cultivating Food Justice: Race, Class, and Sustainability*, edited by Alison Hope Alkon and Julian Agyeman, 89-120. Cambridge, MA: MIT Press.

Minkoff-Zern, Laura-Anne, Nancy Peluso, Jennifer Sowerwine, and Christy Getz. 2011. "Race and Regulation: Asian Immigrants in California Agriculture." In *Cultivating Food Justice: Race, Class, and Sustainability*, edited by Alison Hope Alkon and Julian Agyeman, 65-85. Cambridge, MA: MIT Press.

Morales, Alfonso. 2011. "Growing Food and Justice: Dismantling Racism through Sustainable Food Systems." In *Cultivating*

Food Justice: Race, Class, and Sustainability, edited by Alison Hope Alkon and Julian Agyeman, 149-76. Cambridge, MA: MIT Press.

Norgaard, Kari Mari, Ron Reed, and Carolina Van Horn. 2011. "A Continuing Legacy: Institutional Racism, Hunger, and Nutritional Justice on the Klamath." In *Cultivating Food Justice: Race, Class, and Sustainability*, edited by Alison Hope Alkon and Julian Agyeman, 24-46. Cambridge, MA: MIT Press.

Pollan, Michael. 2008. In *Defense of Food: An Eater's Manifesto*. New York: Penguin.

Rushe, Dominic. 2013. "'Detroit is Basically Broke': Cuts, Cuts, and Cuts to Follow Bankruptcy Filing." *Guardian*, July 19. http://www.theguardian.com/world/2013/jul/19/detroit-broke-bankruptcy.

Runk, David. 2010. "Motor City May Provide Model for Urban Agriculture." *Salon*, April 23. http://www.salon.com/2010/04/23/us_food_and_farm_detroit_farming/

Solnit, Rebecca. 2007. "Detroit Arcadia." *Harper's Magazine*, July, 65-73.

Sugrue, Thomas J. 2005. *The Origins of the Urban Crisis: Race and Inequality in Postwar Detroit*. Princeton: Princeton University Press.

Thompson, Jezra. 2012. "Detroit: Land Grab or City Revival." *Civil Eats*, December 26. http://civileats.com/2012/12/26/detroit-land-grab-or-city-revival/.

Tyner, James A. 2006. "Defend the Ghetto": Space and the Urban Politics of the Black Panther Party." *Annals of the Association of American Geographers* 96 (1): 105-18.

———. 2007. "Urban Revolutions and the Spaces of Black
Radicalism." In *Black Geographies and the Politics of Place*,
edited by Katherine McKittrick and Clyde Woods, 218-32.
Cambridge, MA: South End Press.

US Department of Agriculture. 2009. *Report to Congress: Access
to Affordable and Nutritious Food: Measuring and
Understanding Food Deserts and their Consequences.*
http://www.ers.usda.gov/publications/ap-administrative-
publication/ap-036.aspx#.UVt504V-675.

Voigt, Kate A. 2011. "Pigs in the Backyard or the Barnyard:
Removing Zoning Impediments to Urban Agriculture."
Boston College Environmental Affairs Law Review 38: 537-66.

Ward, Stephen M. 2011. "Introduction to Part IV: Community
Building and Grassroots Leadership in Post-Industrial
Detroit." In *Pages from a Black Radical's Notebook: A James
Boggs Reader,* edited by Stephen M. Ward, 317-21. Detroit,
MI: Wayne State University Press.

Watson, JoAnn. 2013. "THE CITY OF DETROIT HAS NOT FILED
BANKRUPTCY!" *Michigan Citizen*, August 1.
http://michigancitizen.com/the-city-of-detroit-has-not-
filed-bankruptcy/.

White, Monica M. 2010. "Shouldering Responsibility for the
Delivery of Human Rights: A Case of the D-Town Farmers
of Detroit." *Race/Ethnicity: Multidisciplinary Global Contexts* 3
(2): 189-211.

———. 2011a. "D-Town Farm: African American Resistance to
Food Insecurity and the Transformation of Detroit."
Environmental Practice 13 (4): 406-17.

————. 2011b. "Sisters of the Soil: Urban Gardening as Resistance in Detroit." *Race/Ethnicity: Multidisciplinary Global Contexts* 5 (1): 13-28.

Yakini, Malik. 2012a. "A Disturbing Trend." *Be Black and Green* (blog), May 31. http://www.beblackandgreen.com/content/disturbing-trend.

————. 2012b. "What Kind of Urban Farming Will Detroit Have?" *Food First/Institute for Food and Development Policy*, November 30. http://www.foodfirst.org/en/urban+farming+in+Detroit.

————. 2013. "About Us." *Be Black and Green* (blog). Accessed January 23. http://www.beblackandgreen.com/about-us.

Is There a Prescription Drug "Epidemic" in Appalachian Kentucky?: Media Representations and Implications for Women Who Misuse Prescription Drugs

Lesly-Marie Buer

> "Discourse is always harnessed to pull for a social agenda."
> — Otto Santa Ana

Introduction

My dissertation fieldwork will focus on how women navigate treatment for prescription drug misuse in Appalachian Kentucky. Since there is little ethnographic research on prescription drug misuse, drug use in rural areas, or women who use drugs, I examine how the media discusses these issues. The primary purpose of this paper is to analyze how local media sources in Appalachian Kentucky frame prescription drug misuse and women who misuse prescription drugs and the possible implications of these characterizations. I examine articles that were published in 2012 in two local Appalachian Kentucky newspapers from Floyd and Harlan counties. I discuss how Appalachian media discourses are contextualized within national lay and scholarly understandings of drug use and Appalachia. I explain how these media discourses may affect how policies, institutions, and antidrug programs treat those living in Appalachia, especially women who misuse prescription drugs.

Media discourses on those who misuse prescription drugs are important because these discourses both reflect and influence popular imaginings of people who use drugs, people who are deserving of drug treatment or imprisonment, how those who face addiction are healed, and whose health matters. In writing about media representations of women who use drugs, Springer (2010) argues that these popular imaginings in turn affect how private organizations and state and local policy makers understand and deal with women's drug use. For example, Operation Unlawful Narcotics Investigations, Treatment, and Education (UNITE) is a nonprofit organization that works in tandem with local and state officials to combat prescription drug misuse in Appalachian Kentucky. Operation UNITE is widely reported on in the media, and the actions of the organization in turn reflect media discourses on prescription drug misuse. Local media sources may be important in Appalachia because local rather than national sources are more accessible (House and Howard 2009). House and Howard argue that media sources are knowledge gatekeepers who help determine the local agenda by influencing what issues are discussed by the public and the politicians who are garnering public support.

After discussing methods, I focus on two themes that the articles reveal. The columnists and those they quote frame prescription drug misuse as an "epidemic," which connotes a temporal state of exception and casts blame on particular groups, primarily medical providers and drug users. While most articles that blame drug users do not specify gender, I suggest that the articles focused on women who use drugs are more critical. I go on to question the use of the word *epidemic* to describe prescription drug misuse in Appalachian Kentucky. I fully acknowledge that prescription drugs, and prescription pain relievers in particular, are extensively misused in the United States (SAMHSA 2012a). I also understand that OxyContin®, a controlled-release prescription pain reliever, was widely available and misused in Central Appalachia in the 2000s, where there were higher rates of prescriptions for OxyContin as compared to the

United States average (Van Zee 2009). However, *epidemic* is a specific epidemiological term that is being used to characterize prescription drug misuse, and I argue that this terminology may be utilized coercively to maintain structures of power while blaming individuals for drug use. I present possible implications of these media discourses for Appalachian communities and women who misuse prescription drugs. I conclude by calling for further research on media discourses and ethnographic fieldwork on the phenomenon of prescription drug misuse in Appalachia. My discussion of media discourses is nascent and will be expanded upon as I undertake my own ethnographic research.

Methods

I review articles that were published in 2012 in two Appalachian Kentucky newspapers, the *Floyd County Times* based out of Prestonsburg, Kentucky, and the *Harlan Daily Enterprise* based out of Harlan, Kentucky. I used the NewsBank Access World News database to search for articles with the following search terms: *prescription drug*, *pharmaceutical*, *OxyContin*, *drug treatment*, *Suboxone*, *buphrenorphine*, and *methadone*. The search terms that refer to specific prescription drugs were chosen based on my fieldwork in the area. These search terms returned 327 articles. Out of those 327 articles, 158 articles were unique (i.e., not duplicated articles) and relevant to the topic. Irrelevant articles included such topics as access to prescription drugs through the Patient Protection and Affordable Care Act and brief community announcements for drug treatment or fundraising for antidrug programs and institutions. Both articles that originated in the local newspapers' offices and syndicated articles are included. After reading through these articles once and reflecting on literature from anthropology, gender and women's studies, and Appalachian studies, I created a coding scheme and used Dedoose 3.3 to code all articles (SCRC 2012). In terms of citation, while many of the general comments I make refer to my composite analysis of the articles together, I specifically cite newspaper articles I am quoting.

Media Representations

I outline how newspapers and columnists frame prescription drug misuse in Appalachia by giving voice to particular individuals and discuss whom the media blames for prescription drug misuse. State and local columnists and those they quote have labeled prescription drug misuse with a number of scientific and metaphorical descriptors that are meant to scare the public into action, from nine articles calling prescription drug misuse or overdoses from misuse an "epidemic" to a county prosecutor quoted as saying that Appalachian Kentucky is "drowning in a sea of pills" (Kaprowy 2012, A5). Kentucky Governor Steve Beshear has drawn on a variety of metaphors, noting that prescription drug misuse is a "corrosive evil" (Kaprowy 2012, A5), a "scourge" (*FCT* 2012a, A8; *FCT* 2012e, 5A), and a "blight" (*FCT* 2012b, A9).

Most of the individuals who have voice through this set of articles are white, male, and have political power on the local, state, or national level. Those who have voice in these articles are both from within and outside of Appalachian Kentucky and harness the power of scientific terminology to emphasize that they think prescription drug misuse is the primary problem for Kentucky families. In the articles reviewed, the media does not give voice to nonwhite members of the community and those who do not have political power. One of the only women quoted in these articles was Karen Kelly, the director of Operation UNITE, and while Kelly represents one of the few female voices, she is privileged in terms of race, class, and political power.

Three articles focus on the effects of the prescription drug "epidemic" on Kentucky families. Kentucky's Attorney General Jack Conway is quoted as supporting a state House bill that would expand Kentucky's monitoring of prescription drugs because he said the House bill would "save the lives of our friends, our neighbors, and our family members" (*FCT* 2012e, 5A). Governor Beshear espoused a similar idea when he said, "The blight of prescription drug abuse is tearing our families and communities apart, and we must use every tool available to attack this deadly scourge on our state" (*FCT* 2012b, A9). An additional article in the *Floyd County Times* reiterates this point stating that legislation to control prescription drugs will "reduce the destructive impact of prescription drug abuse on Kentucky families" and quoting Kentucky House Speaker Greg Stumbo that legislation "is the most important thing we can do to protect Kentucky families" (*FCT* 2012a, A8). They use the rhetoric of the family and community to conjure nostalgic images of presumably ideal families and communities before the blight of drugs, to generalize the experience of prescription drug misuse, and to therefore justify the "use of every tool available" (*FCT* 2012b, A9) to fight prescription drug misuse.

Although articles invoke Kentucky families to generalize the experience of prescription drug misuse, several columnists and the people they quote use descriptions of prescription drug misuse as an epidemic as a way for them to separate Appalachian Kentucky from the rest of Kentucky. They label Appalachian Kentucky—unlike non-Appalachian Kentucky—as "'ground zero' for the prescription epidemic" (R. Davis 2012b, A1). Scientific terminology is essentially used to "other" Appalachian Kentucky and its inhabitants. For example, Floyd County's prosecutor Brent Turner claims that people outside of Appalachian Kentucky do not understand prescription drug misuse because they are so unlikely to be affected by it (R.

Davis 2012a). Hollywood actors descended on Hazard to perform a play to show the community the harms of prescription drug misuse, which the reporter writes, "prominently affects the Appalachia area" (*FCT* 2012c, A7). One *Floyd County Times* article goes so far as to blame Appalachia for spreading prescription drug misuse to other areas: "Sales of hydrocodone and oxycodone skyrocketed in new parts of the country as the problem spread from its Appalachian roots" (*FCT* 2012d, A8). The columnist Tara Kaprowy's characterization of prescription drug misuse in Kentucky conflates stereotypes of Appalachian Kentuckians with prescription drug misuse:

> Prescription drug abuse has become so prevalent in *parts* of Kentucky, people are buying Mason jars of clean urine at flea markets and under the table at tobacco stores so they can pass drug tests. Kentuckians are pulling out their own teeth so they can go to the dentist to get a three-day prescription for hydrocodone, the most popular pain killer. When they make arrests, law enforcement officers are finding stacks of food stamps that have been traded for pills. Almost two-thirds of Kentuckians have used prescription drugs for non-prescription reasons, 30 percentage points higher than the rest of the country . . . "I think a lot of our people have had enough," said Kerry Harvey, the chief federal prosecutor for Eastern Kentucky. *That's where the problem is worst*, but speakers made clear it is statewide. (Kaprowy 2012, A5; emphasis added)

In Kaprowy's description, prescription drug misusers are turned into foul, toothless, lazy, welfare recipients who spend their food stamps on prescription drugs instead of food. Although Kaprowy acknowledges reports that prescription drug misuse is a statewide problem, she is sure to emphasize that prescription drug misuse is most problematic in Eastern or Appalachian Kentucky. Through these portrayals, Appalachian Kentucky is removed from structural and social contexts and framed as going through an exceptional epidemic, as an exceptional place, and as having an exceptionally foul population.

Although columnists and politicians may use the term *epidemic* to ignore the structural violence present in Appalachia, six articles connected structural inequalities to prescription drug misuse and used their media platform to highlight these inequalities. In a critique of the government's focus on drugs, the local Harlan columnist Bob Franken argues that focusing on drugs is "a good way for them to deflect attention from the real issues, because they can hammer away at drug tests and the other ways they show hostility toward the poor and needy, they don't have to face questions about how it came to be that we have so many who need welfare and unemployment benefits" (Franken 2012, 4). Columnists and some of the politicians they quote associate the following inequalities with prescription drug misuse: labor intensive working conditions, poor roads that cause more motor vehicle accidents, poor environmental conditions, poverty, and lack of access to proper health care and drug treatment.

In terms of who is at fault for the prescription drug epidemic, twenty-five articles blame "rogue" doctors for prescription drug misuse, so according to the compilation of articles, doctors who prescribe too many prescription drugs are most to blame for the "epidemic." One article implicates doctors and the Kentucky Board of Medical Licensure:

> As one former drug trafficking official told reporter RG Dunlop of the apparent toothlessness of the board, "It boils down to this: doctors want to police themselves— and it doesn't work". . . If the licensure board was sketchy in its answers to Courier-Journal questions, Gov. Steve

> Beshear told the newspaper that the board plans to take "swifter, more decisive action" against "drug-dealing doctors who are no longer practicing medicine but who are instead enabling devastating addictions." (*LCJ* 2012a)

In a similar vein, ten articles blame pharmacists for too easily filling prescriptions. I was surprised that only five articles place any culpability on pharmaceutical companies, and the article that most harshly critiques the pharmaceutical industry was written by ProPublica, a nonprofit national investigative journalism organization, and reprinted in the local paper. This dismissal of corporate transgressions and blaming of individual medical providers relates to the use of the term *epidemic* and the exceptionalizing of Appalachia to ignore the social contexts of prescription drug misuse. All of the articles that faulted medical professionals, pharmacists, or the pharmaceutical industry focus on the greed that these misdeeds represented. For the columnists and people they quoted, who were primarily state officials, these villains' actions could be traced to money.

The newspaper articles portray drug users, who are termed *addicts*, as having character flaws beyond just greed, and fifteen articles blame drug users for prescription drug misuse. Drug users are primarily characterized as "doctor shoppers" who are able to dupe multiple doctors into writing prescriptions for pain relievers and as "bad" parents who are exposing their children to the harms of drugs. The following passage exemplifies several articles that are quick to note that in drug arrests of women or coed couples, children were in the same room as prescription drugs and drug paraphernalia: "In the residence, several uncapped needles were located and were in the area creating a risk to two small children that lived in the residence as well . . . the parents of the children were charged with wanton endangerment and endangering the welfare of a minor" (*HDE* 2012,

1). The article assures readers that the children were removed from danger and the parents prosecuted for their actions.

Although more articles focus on blaming addicts generally without specifying gender, the articles that focus on women who misuse prescription drugs are especially critical of mothers and pregnant women for being the medium through which bad science in the form of addictive prescription drugs is socially reproduced through children's exposure and infants' supposed addiction to drugs. For example, an article out of a Louisville newspaper reprinted in the *Harlan Daily Enterprise* blames new mothers who use drugs for all young people's drug and alcohol use (*LCJ* 2012b). Women are also framed as "bad" mothers when they are seen as endangering not only their own children, but all children in the community. One article reiterated multiple times that one woman was caught selling drugs near a high school and was arrested "within view of the Prestonsburg High School" (Latta 2012a, A1).

Another passage exemplifies the articles that blame pregnant women for exposing their newborns to drugs:

> "They are just agitated. They are screaming. Their faces— you have the grimace. They're in pain. Sometimes the babies have seizures." This is a nurse describing what infants look and act like when they are born addicted to drugs. They are the newest and youngest victims of Kentucky's prescription pill epidemic and the number of such infants is growing at an alarming rate . . . Now we learn 730 Kentucky infants were hospitalized last year addicted to drugs, compared to twenty-nine such cases in 2000, and officials blame prescription pill abuse for the skyrocketing numbers. (*LCJ* 2012b)

The scientific authority of the nurse ascribes to infants that are "addicted to drugs" emotions that they cannot directly express, and the columnist ignores other factors that may be causing health problems among infants who are born to marginalized women. The columnist also attributes the increase in rates to increases in prescription drug use, which has actually decreased in Kentucky (SAMHSA 2013), and dismisses other issues that may influence this increase in rates, such as medical providers' greater surveillance of pregnant women. Although the columnist laments that Kentucky does not have more mental health and drug treatment services for pregnant women, they essentially blame pregnant women for reproducing addicted infants: "Clearly the way to stop infants from being born addicted to drugs is to stop pregnant women from drug abuse and addiction" (*LCJ* 2012b).

This columnist, among others, focuses on increasing access to drug treatment for pregnant women and new mothers, reflecting a deeper concern for the actions of pregnant women than for those of nonpregnant women or men. Jack Latta (2012b, 1) celebrates Hope in the Mountains for providing drug treatment to pregnant women and thus protecting infants from drug exposure: "One of the tragic aspects of Eastern Kentucky's drug epidemic is the number of children born into it. Hope in the Mountains offers a place for pregnant women and provides transportation and support to many medical appointments." Drug treatment is generally framed as turning "bad" mothers into "good" mothers by reducing pregnant women's access to "bad" science in the form of prescription drugs, increasing their access to "good" science in the form of drug treatment and prenatal care, getting them jobs, and even teaching them how to garden and cook.

Is this an "epidemic"?

Although the media and political and community leaders draw on scientific authority to make their claims, does the epidemiological research on prescription drug misuse support these statements that Appalachian Kentucky is an epidemic prescription drug war-zone? The CDC defines an *epidemic* as "the occurrence of more cases of disease, injury, or other health condition than expected in a given area or among a specific group of persons during a particular period" (CDC 2007). This definition is somewhat unclear on exactly how many cases of prescription drug misuse should be expected in Appalachian Kentucky. However, comparing rates of prescription drug misuse between Kentucky and other states and within Kentucky indicates that prescription drug misuse is not an epidemic in Appalachian Kentucky in particular. In terms of states with the highest rates of nonmedical use of prescription pain relievers in the past year from 2010 to 2011, Kentucky ranks 31, and rates of nonmedical use of prescription drugs fell in Kentucky from 2009 to 2011 (SAMHSA 2013). Considering regional data on the state of Kentucky, data on rates of nonmedical use of prescription pain relievers in the past year show that misuse of prescription pain relievers was slightly higher in Central and Western Kentucky as compared to Appalachian Kentucky in the years from 2006 to 2010 (SAMHSA 2012b). I grant that these data do have limitations since participants may under- or overexaggerate drug use, and the participants interviewed may not be a representative sample, but there is no evidence that these limitations differ by state or region.

Qualitative research sheds another light on whether or not prescription drug misuse is an epidemic in Appalachian Kentucky. Key informants in one Appalachian Kentucky study stated that prescription drug misuse was not a new phenomenon and that increases in prescription drug misuse were associated with law enforcement's eradication and therefore drug users' decreased use of marijuana in the area (Leukefeld et al. 2007). Agar and Reisinger (2002) similarly show that increases in the use of one type of drug, such as prescription drugs, does not necessarily indicate an epidemic, but a decrease in access to another type of drug, such as heroin. Anglin and White (1999) further complicate the notion of a prescription drug epidemic in Appalachian Kentucky by showing that people in the area go without medication they are prescribed because of expense and that clinicians may misprescribe or overprescribe some prescription drugs because they know that their clients do not have access to mental health services. So why is scientific terminology being appropriated when epidemiological and qualitative research does not support the claims? I provide two possible explanations that will be expanded upon as I gain further understanding of how prescription drug misuse is understood in local communities through my dissertation research.

First, science and scientific terminology connote authority in our society while the media and public equate science with "facts," instead of the context in which science is produced (Martin 1987). Using the public health terminology of an *epidemic* gives these speakers authority to "use every tool available," in the words of Governor Beshear (*FCT* 2012a, A8), to fix the problem of prescription drug misuse in Appalachian Kentucky, whether that is by reforming the Appalachian family, removing children from the care of parents, or sending individuals who misuse prescription drugs to mandatory drug treatment or jail. Warwick Anderson (2006) reminds us that the state exerts power over the population, especially the marginalized or those deemed dangerous, in the name of public health. Although "well-meaning people" may cling to terms such as *epidemic* to fight perceived public health threats, they, unknowingly or not, utilize public health in the public "damning" of marginalized populations and rationalization of social inequality in order to maintain their own cultural dominance and privilege (Geronimus 2003, 882).

In the articles reviewed, the term *epidemic* connotes a temporal state of exception where state officials, of whom the vast majority are male and all are white and elite, are given power to restructure the law, families, and individuals in Appalachian Kentucky. Although those who are privileged by gender, race, and class may instigate the discourse used to discuss this state of exception, this discourse becomes part of everyday common knowledge, is no longer used by only those with privileged positions, and may be employed to control even those who enjoy privileged positions. In other words, the epidemic that is the temporal state of exception expands beyond the creators and comes to discipline the entire population, although those who are less privileged are more intensely surveyed and face more damaging consequences when they are disciplined. "Appalachia" as a discursive construction connotes a geographic state of exception that is framed as spatially as well as culturally separated from the rest of the United States. As shown through the examples presented in this paper and previous academic analyses, media sources, policy makers, and scholars have often stereotyped Appalachians as foul, toothless, and lazy, and as drains on social spending (Billings 2008; Scott 2010; see Ford 1967). According to Agamben (1998), a state of exception occurs in an excluded area during a political, economic, or health crisis where the state assumes more power than usual in order to maintain the status quo and the state continues to exert this power even after the crisis is over. Through media discourses on prescription drug misuse in Appalachia, people in Appalachia who misuse prescription drugs are removed from political life and "the qualified life of the citizen" through the dismissal of political and structural factors that may affect drug use and the marginalization of drug users (Agamben 1998, 73). Through the use of the term *epidemic* to render Appalachia an exceptional place in the middle of an exceptional time, Appalachian women's lives in particular are rendered as bare life and prime for the state's implementation of biopolitics.

Second, using the epidemiological terminology of an *epidemic* allows most media sources to ignore social factors that are contributing to prescription drug misuse, such as structural violence. Paul Farmer (1999, 2003) understands structural violence as encompassing a number of different mechanisms that lead to the uneven distribution of human suffering and operate through institutions and social environments. Lutz and Nonini (1999) connect structural violence to the systematic marginalization and exploitation of labor through capitalism, and D. Davis (2004) ties structural violence to neoliberal policies that remove the social safety net for those in poverty and thus limit people's access to resources. Public health literature has associated poor labor conditions, which cause higher rates of workplace injuries, high rates of poverty and unemployment, and lack of medically appropriate pain and drug treatment with illicit drug use in rural areas (Dew, Elifson, and Dozier 2007; Passik 2003). However, the media generally frames "Appalachianess" as an individual risk factor for prescription drug misuse instead of connecting the structural violence in Appalachia to prescription drug misuse.

Although the coal industry is rarely demonized in Appalachian media sources, the coal industry is connected to structural violence because it exploits labor economically and physically, pollutes the environment, and exacerbates social inequalities based on gender because men are associated with coal mining jobs (House and Howard 2009; Scott 2010). The coal industry's war against unions is related to increasingly exploitive and unsafe labor conditions and miners' decreased access to employee health insurance and health care programs (Anglin and White 1999; McNeil 2005). Decreased numbers of coal mining jobs in the region, largely due to increasing mechanization and more intrusive mining processes, such as mountaintop removal, exacerbate unemployment, poverty, and lack of access to health care (Anglin and White 1999; McNeil 2005). The coal industry is directly implicated in prescription drug misuse as unsafe labor conditions lead to injuries that are treated by addictive prescription pain relievers, and key informants in Appalachia have indicated that coal companies are quicker to provide injured employees prescription pain relievers rather than costly medical procedures that may permanently alleviate pain (Anglin and White 1999). However, media sources deflect attention away from the most detrimental impacts of the coal industry. In 2012, although the two newspaper sources cited in this paper printed 158 articles regarding prescription drug misuse, only nine articles were printed about mountaintop removal, and two of those nine articles claimed that anti-mountaintop removal activists were launching a "war on coal." Blaming only individuals for drug use while dismissing social or structural issues is characteristic of neoliberalism (Ortiz and Briggs 2003; Springer 2010) and mainstream epidemiology (Krieger 2011; Inhorn and Whittle 2001).

Haraway (1989), drawing on Foucault, understands power and domination as not things that are simply possessed, but as things that are exercised through the continual production of knowledge. Using Haraway's (1989) concept of power, producing the knowledge of prescription drug misuse as an epidemic and as the primary problem of a region allows those who benefit from the hierarchal social order in the area to maintain structures of domination. By focusing on battling the epidemic, columnists and politicians generally ignore the association of women's drug use with the feminization of poverty, domestic violence, and increased homelessness among women (Chavkin and Breitbart 1997). On the other hand, Haraway (1989) notes that discourse can be used to both maintain and weaken structures of domination. Columnists like Franken (2012) use discourse to bring attention to the inequalities he sees. Further, labeling Appalachian Kentucky as having an "epidemic" may help politicians and local leaders funnel needed resources into the area for a wide variety of uses that could be beneficial, from creating after-school programs to providing drug treatment to women.

Specific Implications for Women

I discuss how who has voice in the media and how media portrayals of prescription drug misuse may affect how society, policies, and institutions treat women who misuse prescription drugs. While feminist science studies asks us to examine who is allowed to speak and who has access to knowledge (Rouse 1996), the fact that Karen Kelly was one of the only women quoted in the articles shows that we must also consider how those who have been silenced in the past use the authority of science to gain voice and who these formally marginalized voices in turn silence. For example, white middle-class women in the United States used domestic science to enter into professions outside of the home, such as social work and nursing, in the late nineteenth and early twentieth centuries (Tomes 1998). Tomes (1998) argues that this move by white middle-class women advanced their class and racial interests by providing a space for middle-class women's political involvement and reasserting Anglo-American cultural dominance over immigrant groups. In Appalachia during the same time period, middle- and upper-class white women, a group in which Karen Kelly is now a member, joined voluntary organizations that advocated scientific medicine and associated with male physicians in order to gain some autonomy in the public sphere (Barney 2000). Although Kelly is one of the only women quoted in these newspaper articles, she is privileged because she is white and middle to upper class. I suggest that all of the speakers, unintentionally or not, use their differing levels of privilege to degrade and discipline those who are not associated with white middle-class norms.

The implementation of biopolitics on the lives of Appalachian women is supported by the historic use of domestic science, public health, and reproductive technologies. I argue that framing prescription drug misuse as an epidemic and incriminating Kentucky families, particularly Appalachian Kentucky families, has gendered implications. Although men may be framed as being financially responsible for the well-being of the family in the United States and Appalachia specifically (Scott 2010), women are framed as being responsible for the moral, emotional, and physical health of the family (Barney 2000; Becker 1998; Tomes 1998) and thus more at fault for substance use. In other words, when the media implicates families as fostering or being the victims of substance abuse, women, especially mothers, are the absent referent. The state has used its power with discursive and material support from public health and private citizens to try to transform the "pathological" Appalachian family through the implementation of domestic science. The state supported middle-class women's volunteer groups and settlement houses in the 1930s in Appalachia that aimed to transform poor women's behaviors and thus the lives of working-class families (Barney 2000). Poor women in coal mining camps were seen to be responsible for their family's health, and middle-class women backed by male physicians encouraged poor women to cling to the ideals of scientific medicine in order to lift their families out of poverty (Barney 2000). These developments in Appalachia paralleled similar efforts across the United States during this time period (Tomes 1998).

Feminist writings connect the representation of women who use drugs in Appalachia to society-wide representations in the United States. Mothers who use drugs challenge "good" mother ideals and are thus stigmatized (Goodwin 2011; Whiteford and Vitucci 1997).

The ideal mother is supposed to be "sexually virtuous, self-sacrificing, nurturing, and drug-free" (Bourgois and Schonberg 2009, 207). The media and policy makers portray women who use drugs as "bad" mothers because they are framed as putting their children's health at risk in "their reckless search for pleasure" (Flavin and Paltrow 2010, 232; Whiteford and Vitucci 1997). According to Baker and Carson (1999, 349), the United States national media frames women who use drugs as "bad" mothers and, "any substance-abusing woman is invariably a 'bad' mother, for it is assumed that the search for, and the use of, substances makes her inattentive, self-indulgent, and negligent rather [than] exclusively mindful of her children's needs."

Notions of "ideal" motherhood intersect with gender, race, and class to shape how some women are framed as "bad" mothers. "Ideal" motherhood in the United States is defined by "white, heterosexual, married, middle-class" norms (Flavin 2009, chap. 7). Single mothers, mothers of color, and mothers who fall outside of the middle class violate these norms and risk being labeled as "bad" mothers (Flavin 2009). The first prosecutions of pregnant women and mothers who tested positive for drugs in the 1980s reflect issues of ideal motherhood and race (Roberts 1997; Whiteford and Vitucci 1997). Mothers of so-called "crack babies" were defined as "bad" mothers because they were assumed to be "promiscuous, uncaring, and self-indulgent," the opposite of what an ideal mother should be (Flavin and Paltrow 2010; Roberts 1997, 156). Mothers of "crack babies" were also assumed to be black and associated with other stigmatized caricatures of black mothers, such as matriarchs and "welfare queens" (Reagan 2010; Roberts 1997).

Although how the state uses public health may affect everyone to some degree, it has specific implications for marginalized women who are labeled as "bad" mothers. The state has used the science of public health to justify the forced or coerced sterilization of poor women, women of color, women who use drugs, and Appalachian women (Briggs 2002; A. Davis 1990; Lock and Nguyen 2010; Nelson 2003; Roberts 1997; Smith 2005). In the name of public health, private organizations have joined the state in funding and promoting sterilizations for women who use drugs. For instance, Project Prevention is a private initiative that began in the 1990s in North Carolina and targets primarily low-income women of color who use drugs in order to pay them $300 to become sterilized or to use long-acting contraceptives (Lucke and Hall 2012; Silliman et al. 2004). Project Prevention, which has spread from North Carolina to communities across the United States and United Kingdom, was originally called Children Requiring Caring Communities (CRACK) (Project Prevention 2013; Silliman et al. 2004), and quite obviously plays off of the "crack baby" fears that originated in the 1980s (see Ortiz and Briggs 2003). Barbara Harris, the founder, uses the "concerned mother" tactic to garner support for her organization claiming that she founded CRACK because she adopted children from an addicted mother and saw these children struggle through life (Project Prevention 2013; see Mason 2009). The organization claims that its goal is to reduce the number of infants who are exposed to illicit drugs (Lucke and Hall 2012), but the organization overemphasizes the effects of illicit drugs on fetal health and ignores the effects that legal drugs may have on fetal health (see Chavkin and Breitbart 1997).

State policies have served to jail or civilly commit women while they were pregnant in an effort to stop their drug use, have temporarily or permanently terminated using women's parental rights, and have prosecuted women for using drugs while pregnant (Paltrow 2000; Roberts 1997). Criminal charges started being brought against pregnant women who tested positive for drugs in the 1980s when there was a rise in public fear over "crack babies" (Roberts 1997).

Hundreds of women in forty states have been arrested while they were pregnant because they were identified as drug users (Flavin and Paltrow 2010). When these prosecutions have been challenged, they have been overturned in every state but South Carolina (Flavin and Paltrow 2010). In South Carolina in 1992, Cornelia Whitner was one of the first women to be convicted of unlawful child neglect based on her alleged drug use during pregnancy (Chavkin and Breitbart 1997; Paltrow 2000). Although the infant was in good health when born, Whitner was still prosecuted because trace amounts of cocaine were found in the infant's urine (Roberts 1997). The civil and criminal punishments inflicted on women are often based on the premise that "fetal rights" are separate from mother's rights and that the interests of the fetus are equal to or greater than the interests of the pregnant woman (Flavin 2009; Paltrow 2000; Roberts 1997).

Reagan (2010) agrees that initial prosecutions of pregnant women targeted low-income women of color but shows how prosecutions have been expanded to include drug users who are assumed to be white, poor, unemployed, and located in rural America. She argues that prosecutions of poor white women demonstrate that class may be as important as gender and race in determining which women society targets and frames as "bad" mothers (Reagan 2010). The media, society, and prosecutors target low-income women for prosecution in their stigmatization of mothers who use drugs. Women receiving care at publicly funded hospitals are often screened for drugs, making it more likely that they will be reported to government officials (Whiteford and Vitucci 1997). However, clients receiving care from private hospitals are rarely screened for drugs because clinicians are afraid they will lose the business of clients if they do screen them (Whiteford and Vitucci 1997). Thus, women who can afford to go to private hospitals or doctors are less likely to be reported to government officials for testing positive for drug use during pregnancy as compared to poor women who are more likely to rely on public health care (Springer 2010). In one study, most of the women targeted by state intervention were poor or working class because women who were privileged according to class were less likely to have to come into contact with or rely on welfare and human service bureaucracies to survive financially (Baker and Carson 1999).

Federal authorities, such as Henry Vaughn of the Tennessee Valley Authority, have historically characterized Appalachian women as uncivilized "beasts of burden" to justify federal development of Appalachian lands and the implementation of biopolitics on Appalachian women's bodies (Becker 1998). Coercive promotion of contraception and sterilization is not new in Appalachia, where Clarence Gamble developed several programs to reduce the number of children Appalachian women had in the 1930s (Briggs 2002). Gamble's US programs were primarily located in Appalachia—Kentucky, North Carolina, Tennessee, Virginia, and West Virginia—with Florida having the only program outside of the region (Briggs 2002). Gamble was not concerned with whether or not the programs he promoted served the needs of local women or if women even wanted the programs (Briggs 2002). He claimed that reduced fertility among working-class women would end poverty, increase the intellectual capacity of the country, and ultimately maintain the modern social structure (Briggs 2002).

The media, public officials, and clinicians continue to espouse misinformation using claims to science about the effects of illicit substance use on fetuses, especially use of crack and methamphetamine (Flavin and Paltrow 2010; Reagan 2010; see Sterk 1999). However, the effects of illicit substance use on fetal health and child health are unclear (Chavkin and Breitbart 1997; Flavin 2009). Policies that punish pregnant women overemphasize the health risks associated with drug consumption to fetuses and completely dismiss the health of women (Flavin and Paltrow 2010). Policy makers and media sources ignore the environment in which women live and the possible effects of this environment on the health of women, fetuses, and children (Flavin and Paltrow 2010; Reagan 2010; Whiteford and Vitucci 1997). Women who use illicit drugs are more likely to be poor, sick, physically abused, and to lack prenatal care (Goodwin 2011; Roberts 1997). Policies that punish pregnant women or provide medical care and drug treatment only to pregnant women promote injustice because society expects a pregnant woman to give her fetus access to health care and a healthy environment that she does not even have access to (Flavin and Paltrow 2010). Further, these policies ignore the effects that legal drugs, such as tobacco and alcohol, may have on women's health, fetal development, and child health, perhaps because these drugs are more often associated with white and/or wealthier women (Baker and Carson 1999; Paltrow 2000).

Although I critique the media for exceptionalizing Appalachian women, I take from feminist theory a wariness of either concentrating on specificities or generalities. Both focusing on the particularities of women's experiences of prescription drug misuse in Appalachian Kentucky and on the generalities of women's experiences of drug use nationally or globally ignore or silence others (Harris 1990). The first focus ignores the fact that there are many women who experience substance abuse, and the second focus ignores the fact that women experience substance abuse in more than one way based on a host of individual and structural factors. Harris (1990, 586) argues that focusing on particularities prevents "moral responsibility or social change," but recommends that feminists continue to see categories and generalizations as "tentative, relational, and unstable." Labeling women's prescription drug misuse as an "Appalachian" problem may absolve the media from discussing structural violence in the region, but trying to show that prescription drug misuse happens everywhere may take the focus off the very real problems of prescription drug use and lack of access to appropriate health care in Appalachia.

Conclusion

Through this paper, I have shown how the media depicts prescription drug misuse in Appalachian Kentucky and suggest how this characterization may serve the interests of those in power. By calling prescription drug misuse an epidemic and making Appalachia seem like an exceptional place, politicians and policy makers bolster their power to change Appalachian families and women through state interference. Although I critique the exceptionalism of Appalachia, we should not ignore the particular circumstances that may surround drug use in Appalachia and that the labeling of Appalachia as exceptional has economic implications in terms of federal and state funding.

The focus on prescription drug misuse as the only problem in Appalachian Kentucky absolves politicians, columnists, and society from any complicity they may have in supporting mechanisms of structural violence in Appalachian Kentucky. Through blaming "rogue" medical providers and "bad" mothers for prescription drug misuse, the media again absolves society or corporations from any wrongdoing. They reflect sexist, racist, and classist understandings of drug use that have implications for women who use drugs as women are expected to give their families, children, and fetuses access to more resources than they themselves have access to.

There are certainly limitations to this study because it focuses on only two newspapers in the region for a one-year time span. In order to more fully grasp how the media frames prescription drug misuse in Appalachia, additional regional and national news sources should be examined. Further research also needs to be done in Appalachia regarding prescription drug misuse. For example, how does the media affect who the public thinks is worthy of being healed? How are state and local initiatives to combat prescription drug misuse affecting women's everyday lives? How is structural violence connected to women's drug use in Appalachian Kentucky? How do women embody characterizations of women who use drugs, and how do these characterizations affect their access to drug treatment?

Works Cited

Agamben, Giorgio. 1998. *Homo Sacer: Sovereign Power and Bare Life*. Stanford, CA: Stanford University Press.

Agar, Michael, and Heather Schacht Reisinger. 2002. "A Tale of Two Policies: The French Connection, Methadone, and Heroin Epidemics." *Culture, Medicine, and Psychiatry* 26 (3): 371-96.

Anderson, Warwick. 2006. *Colonial Pathologies: American Tropical Medicine, Race, and Hygiene in the Philippines*. Durham, NC: Duke University Press.

Anglin, Mary K., and Jill Collins White. 1999. "Poverty, Health Care, and Problems of Prescription Medication: A Case Study." *Substance Use and Misuse* 34 (14): 2073-93.

Baker, Phyllis L., and Amy Carson. 1999. "'I Take Care of My Kids': Mothering Practices of Substance-Abusing Women." *Gender and Society* 13 (3): 347-63.

Barney, Sandra Lee. 2000. *Authorized to Health: Gender, Class, and the Transformation of Medicine in Appalachia, 1880-1930*. Chapel Hill: University of North Carolina Press.

Becker, Jane S. 1998. *Selling Tradition: Appalachia and the Construction of an American Folk 1930-1940*. Chapel Hill: University of North Carolina Press.

Billings, Dwight. 2008. "Economic Representations in an American Region: What's at Stake in Appalachia?" In *Economic Representation: Economic and Everyday*, edited by David F. Ruccio, 156-69. New York: Routledge.

Bourgois, Philippe, and Jeff Schonberg. 2009. *Righteous Dopefiend*. Berkeley: University of California Press.

Briggs, Laura. 2002. *Reproducing Empire: Race, Sex, Science, and US Imperialism in Puerto Rico*. Berkeley: University of California Press.

CDC (Centers for Disease Control). 2007. "Glossary of Epidemiology Terms." http:// www.cdc.gov/excite/library/glossary.htm.

Chavkin, Wendy, and Vicki Breitbart. 1997. "Substance Abuse and Maternity: The United States as a Case Study." *Addiction* 92 (9): 1201-5.

Davis, Angela. 1990. "Racism, Birth Control, and Reproductive Rights." In *Abortion Rights to Reproductive Freedom: Transforming a Movement*, edited by Marlene Fried, 15-26. Boston, MA: South End Press.

Davis, Dana-Ain. 2004. "Manufacturing Mammies: The Burdens of Service Work and Welfare Reform among Battered Black Women." *Anthropologica* 46 (2): 273-88.

Davis, Ralph B. 2012a. "Turner Part of State Pill Summit." *Floyd County Times*, January 25:A1.

————. 2012b. "Leaders Discuss Drug Problem." *Floyd County Times*, October 31:A1.

Dew, Brian, Kirk Elifson, and Michael Dozier. 2007. "Social and Environmental Factors and Their Influence on Drug Use Vulnerability and Resiliency in Rural Populations." *Journal of Rural Health* 23 Supplement: S16-21.

Farmer, Paul. 1999. *Infections and Inequalities: The New Modern Plagues*. Berkeley: University of California Press.

————. 2003. *Pathologies of Power: Health, Human Rights, and the New War on the Poor*. Berkeley: University of California Press.

Flavin, Jeanne. 2009. *Our Bodies, Our Crimes: The Policing of Women's Reproduction in America*. Kindle Edition. New York: New York University Press.

_____, and Lynn M. Paltrow. 2010. "Punishing Pregnant Drug-Using Women: Defying Law, Medicine, and Common Sense." *Journal of Addictive Diseases* 29 (2): 231-44.

FCT (Floyd County Times). 2012a. "Governor Support Drug Bills by Stumbo, Others." February 8:A8.

_____. 2012b. "Kentucky Joins Program to Share Prescription Data." March 30:A9.

_____. 2012c. "Addiction Takes Center Stage—Panel Discussion, Public Forum to Address Local Solutions." April 6:A7.

_____. 2012d. "Pain-Pill Problem has Spread to New Areas from Appalachia." April 11:A8.

_____. 2012e. "4 Pain Clinics Close After Pill Bill Takes Effect." July 27:5A.

Ford, Thomas R. 1967. *The Southern Appalachian Region: A Survey*. Lexington: University of Kentucky Press.

Franken, Bob. 2012. "Turning Our Focus to the Drug Fix." *Harlan Daily Enterprise*, March 3:4.

Geronimus, Arline T. 2003. "Damned If You Do: Culture, Identity, Privilege, and Teenage Childbearing in the United States." *Social Science and Medicine* 57 (5): 881-93.

Goodwin, Michele Bratcher. 2011. "Precarious Moorings: Tying Fetal Drug Law Policy to Social Profiling." *Rutgers Law Journal* 42:659-94.

Haraway, Donna. 1989. *Primate Visions: Gender, Race, and Nature in the World of Modern Science*. New York: Routledge.

Harris, Angela P. 1990. "Race and Essentialism in Feminist Legal Theory." *Stanford Law Review* 42 (3): 581-616.

HDE (Harlan Daily Enterprise). 2012. "Deputies Conduct Raid at Sawbrair—Evarts Man Sentenced in Bell Co." October 13:1.

House, Silas, and Jason Howard. 2009. "Introduction." In *Something's Rising: Appalachians Fighting Mountaintop Removal*, edited by Silas House and Jason Howard, 1-21. Lexington: University Press of Kentucky.

Inhorn, Marcia C., and K. Lisa Whittle. 2001. "Feminism Meets the 'New' Epidemiologies: Toward an Appraisal of Antifeminist Biases in Epidemiological Research on Women's Health." *Social Science and Medicine* 53 (5): 553-67.

Kaprowy, Tara. 2012. "Shocking Realities of Prescription Pill Abuse Drive another Summit to Get Everyone in Harness to Fight It." *Floyd County Times*, February 3:A5.

Krieger, Nancy. 2011. *Epidemiology and the People's Health: Theory and Context*. New York: Oxford University Press.

Latta, Jack. 2012a. "One Woman Arrested after Drug Buy." *Floyd County Times*, March 2:A1.

————. 2012b "Growing Hope—Women's Treatment Center Growing Fourfold." *Floyd County Times*, May 25:1.

LCJ (*Louisville Courier-Journal*). 2012a. "Drug Series Aims Toward Reform Need." *Harlan Daily Enterprise*, January 5.

————. 2012b. "Plan of Attack Needed for Drug-Addicted Newborns." *Harlan Daily Enterprise*, September 8.

Leukefeld, Carl, Robert Walker, Jennifer Havens, Cynthia A. Leedham, and Valarie Tolbert. 2007. "What Does the Community Say: Key Informant Perceptions of Rural Prescription Drug Use." *Journal of Drug Issues* 37 (3): 503-24.

Lock, Margaret, and Vinh-Kim Nguyen. 2010. *An Anthropology of Biomedicine*. Malden, MA: Wiley-Blackwell.

Lucke, Jayne C., and Wayne D. Hall. 2012. "Under What Conditions is it Ethical to Offer Incentives to Encourage Drug-Using

Women to Use Long-Acting Forms of Contraception?" *Addiction* 107 (6): 1036-41.

Lutz, Catherine, and Donald Nonini. 1999. "The Economies of Violence and the Violence of Economies." In *Anthropological Theory Today*, edited by Henrietta L. Moore, 73-113. Malden, MA: Polity Press.

Martin, Emily. 1987. *The Woman in the Body: A Cultural Analysis of Reproduction*. Boston, MA: Beacon Press.

Mason, Carol. 2009. *Reading Appalachia from Left to Right: Conservatives and the 1974 Kanawha County Textbook Controversy*. Ithaca, NY: Cornell University Press.

McNeil, Bryan. 2005. "Global Forces, Local Worlds: Mountaintop Removal and Appalachian Communities." In *The American South in a Global World*, edited by James L. Peacock, Harry L. Watson, and Carrie R. Matthews, 99-110. Chapel Hill: University of North Carolina Press.

Nelson, Jennifer. 2003. *Women of Color and the Reproductive Rights Movement*. New York: New York University Press.

Ortiz, Ana Teresa, and Laura Briggs. 2003. "The Culture of Poverty, Crack Babies, and Welfare Cheats: The Making of the 'Healthy White Baby Crisis.'" *Social Text* 21 (3): 39-57.

Paltrow, Lynn. 2000. *Punishing Women for Their Behavior during Pregnancy: An Approach That Undermines Women's Health and Children's Interests*. New York: Center for Reproductive Rights.

Passik, Steven D. 2003. "Same as It Ever Was? Life after the OxyContin Frenzy." *Journal of Pain and Symptom Management* 25 (3): 199-201.

Project Prevention. 2013. "Project Prevention: Frequently Asked Questions." http://www.projectprevention.org/faq/.

Reagan, Leslie J. 2010. *Dangerous Pregnancies: Mothers, Disabilities, and Abortion in Modern America*. Berkeley: University of California Press.

Roberts, Dorothy. 1997. *Killing the Black Body: Race Reproduction and the Meaning of Liberty*. New York: Pantheon Books.

Rouse, Joseph. 1996. "Feminism and the Social Construction of Scientific Knowledge." In *Feminism, Science, and the Philosophy of Science*, edited by Lynn Hankinson Nelson, 195-215. Norwell: Kluwer Academic Publishers.

SAMHSA (Substance Abuse and Mental Health Services Administration). 2012a. Results from the 2011 National Survey on Drug Use and Health: Summary of National Findings. Rockville, MD: Center for Behavioral Health Statistics and Quality.

————. 2012b. *National Survey on Drug Use and Health: Comparison of the 2006-2008 and 2008-2010 Model-Based Substate Estimates*. Rockville, MD: Center for Behavioral Health Statistics and Quality.

————. 2013. *The NSDUH Report: State Estimates of Nonmedical Use of Prescription Pain Relievers*. Rockville, MD: Center for Behavioral Health Statistics and Quality.

Santa Ana, Otto. 2002. *Brown Tide Rising: Metaphors of Latinos in Contemporary American Public Discourse*. Austin: University of Texas Press.

Scott, Rebecca. 2010. *Removing Mountains: Extracting Nature and Identity in the Appalachian Coalfields*. Kindle Edition. Minneapolis: University of Minnesota Press.

SCRC (SocioCultural Research Consultants). 2012. Dedoose 3.3. Los Angeles, CA: SocioCultural Research Consultants, LLC.

Silliman, Jael, Marlene Gerber Fried, Loretta Ross, and Elena
        Gutierrez. 2004. *Undivided Rights: Women of Color
        Organizing for Reproductive Justice*. Cambridge, MA: South
        End Press.

Smith, Andrea. 2005. *Conquest: Sexual Violence and American
        Indian Genocide*. Boston, MA: South End Press.

Springer, Kristen W. 2010. "The Race and Class Privilege of
        Motherhood: The New York Times Presentations of
        Pregnant Drug-Using Women." *Sociological Forum* 25 (3):
        476-99.

Sterk, Claire E. 1999. *Fast Lives: Women Who Use Crack Cocaine*.
        Philadelphia, PA: Temple University Press.

Tomes, Nancy. 1998. *The Gospel of Germs: Men, Women, and
        the Microbe in American Life*. Cambridge, MA: Harvard
        University Press.

Van Zee, Art. 2009. "The Promotion and Marketing of OxyContin:
        Commercial Triumph, Public Health Tragedy." *American
        Journal of Public Health* 99 (2): 221-27.

Whiteford, Linda M., and Judi Vitucci. 1997. "Pregnancy and
        Addiction: Translating Research into Practice." *Social
        Science and Medicine* 44 (9): 1371-80.

Acknowledgments

I would like to thank Dr. Melissa Stein from the University of Kentucky's Department of Gender and Women's Studies and Henry Bundy from the University of Kentucky's Department of Anthropology for commenting on previous drafts of this paper.

The Cultural Context of Depression in Appalachia: Evangelical Christianity and the Experience of Emotional Distress and Healing

Susan E. Keefe and Lisa Curtin

Survey research by Zhang et al. (2008) found that Appalachian residents report experiencing a greater prevalence of serious psychological distress compared to non-Appalachian residents. Specifically, Appalachians report a significantly higher prevalence of major depressive episodes compared to non-Appalachians. Locally conducted studies in Appalachia also find high rates of depression among residents (Hauenstein and Peddada 2007; Huttlinger, Schaller-Ayers, and Lawson 2004; Mutaner and Barnett 2000). Other studies suggest that Appalachian natives are at high risk for suicide, which is often associated with depression (Halverson, Ma, and Harner 2004). We assume that stressors such as high rates of unemployment and poverty, low levels of education and health insurance coverage, long distances to services, fewer institutional resources, and cultural differences between clients and service providers increase the prevalence of mental and emotional problems such as depression in the region. Despite higher rates of depression and suicide, there is little evidence of a higher demand for mental health services in Appalachia. Neither has there been much research on the experience of depression among Appalachian natives.

In 2011, we began a research project investigating illness narratives among Appalachians experiencing depression. We used medical anthropologist Arthur Kleinman's (1980) suggested interview guide for understanding the patient's experience of illness (as opposed to the biomedical definition of diseases). The questions cover five major topics: etiology, time and mode of onset of symptoms, pathophysiology, course of sickness, and treatment. Our intent was to begin to understand the psychosocial experience and the meaning of depression as perceived by Appalachian natives. We decided to begin with a sample of individuals who had been diagnosed with depression or who were taking antidepressants. Following confidentiality requirements, we solicited volunteers from the offices of physicians, clinics, mental health professionals, and peer support groups in two rural counties in western North Carolina. We offered a stipend of $50 if participants completed all forms and an in-person interview. We distributed 450 flyers over six months. We anticipated receiving a large response. After considerable effort, we received a total of thirty-seven volunteers for the study. After screening for native birthplace and diagnosis, however, we were left with a sample of only twenty-three consultants in the final interviews.

Not only did we have difficulty in gathering a sample, but the final sample appears to be unusual in many ways. Most of our consultants have had severe symptoms. Many have been suffering for decades, requiring repeated hospitalizations, often for suicide attempts. Several have psychological symptoms so severe they have qualified for and are living on disability. Many experience comorbidity with anxiety, alcohol abuse, PTSD or other psychological disorders, or with chronic physical health problems.

Given the high rate of depression in Appalachia, this paper attempts to make sense of the problems we had in attracting a larger sample with a range of symptoms from mild cases to more severe. We begin by briefly introducing the current biopsychosocial model of the symptoms, etiology, and treatment of depression utilized by mental health professionals. Then we move to an examination of the cultural context of rural Appalachia, particularly the religious nature of evangelical Christianity and culturally embedded conceptions of emotional distress as well as appropriate healing. A case study provides insight into the cultural context for one individual from our sample who suffers from depression.

Symptoms, Etiology, and Treatment of Depression According to Mental Health Professionals

Depression is typically defined using the objective diagnostic criteria specified in the Diagnostic and Statistical Manual of Mental Disorders (e.g., DSM-5; American Psychiatric Association 2013) or the International Statistical Classification of Diseases and Related Health Problems-10 (World Health Organization 1992). Depression, as a syndrome, is defined by depressed mood and/or a lack of pleasure in addition to a host of related symptoms including profound loss of interest in activities, appetite and sleep disturbance, feelings of guilt and worthlessness, changes in behavior, and potentially suicidal ideation and impulses across a minimum of two weeks in the absence of mania. Depression is considered a leading cause of disability worldwide and a treatable illness.

Medicine and psychology offer numerous etiological conceptualizations of depression, but most employ a diathesis-stress model to understand an individual's depression (Beck 1979; Lazarus 1993). A diathesis-stress model accounts for predisposing vulnerabilities, such as a positive family history of depression and dysfunctional attitudes (e.g., negative attitudes toward self, others, and future) as well as negative life events that oftentimes precede and trigger depression (Abela & D'Alessandro 2002). Most modern perspectives on depression, as well as other illnesses, deviate from a pure biomedical model and consider biological, psychological, and social factors as important in the etiology and maintenance of the disorder (Engel 1977). Thus, vulnerabilities to depression differ from person to person and may be genetic, biological (e.g., serotonin dysfunction), psychological (e.g., personality, learning experiences, internalized messages), or social (e.g., early negative experiences) in nature (Savaneau and Nemeroff 2012). In addition, biological, psychological, and social variables are not considered in isolation but are considered interdependent. In turn, most practitioners employ an idiosyncratic method of case conceptualization and treatment based on a thorough assessment of an individual client's symptomology, vulnerabilities, current stressors, and strengths (e.g., coping skills, social support, economic resources).

Ideally, psychotherapy is evidence-based and individualized with attention to cultural context rather than a one-size-fits-all approach (American Psychological Association 2012). Indeed, psychotherapy, particularly cognitive-behavioral therapy that focuses on increasing engagement in reinforcing behaviors and challenging irrational and self-defeating thoughts, has been found to be as effective as medication in the treatment of depression (Antonuccio, Danton, and DeNelsky 1995). However, between 1998 and 2007, the use of psychotropic medications for the outpatient treatment of mental illness increased, and the average number of outpatient psychotherapy sessions decreased (Olfson and Marcus 2010). In addition, there is concern about the potential for increased use of antidepressant medications for the treatment of depression in the future. For example, the DSM-5 allows for the diagnosis of Major Depression in the context of bereavement whereas the DSM-IV did not unless symptoms persisted longer than two months or resulted in significant impairment. Many practitioners and researchers (e.g., Friedman 2012) are concerned that this diagnostic change may pathologize the normal process of grief and that unnecessary intervention, particularly the use of antidepressants, could interfere with adaptation to loss and grief.

"It's a weakness, not an illness": A Case Study

The following case study collected during our research presents an Appalachian response to depression. Sammy's experience illustrates that evangelical Christians have a different way of interpreting the symptoms and etiology of emotional suffering ascribed to depression in the biopsychosocial model just described.

Sammy[1] is a forty-eight-year-old woman who grew up in a rural part of a nearby county. Sammy's father was a Baptist preacher. He never had his own church, in part because he got divorced, which is considered a sin among conservative evangelical Christians. He has had a brain aneurism in recent years and was diagnosed with depression and schizophrenia as a result of that, according to Sammy. Her mother suffered from depression, was suicidal, and had nervous breakdowns many times; she often left young Sammy to fend for herself beginning when Sammy was a preschooler. When her parents were separating and her mother was drinking, Sammy became the object of their anger and violence. Sammy tried to commit suicide and was hospitalized at the age of eighteen. Her father refused to take her to counseling afterwards, according to Sammy, because he was ashamed.

Sammy proceeded to give a detailed portrait of how religion in the mountains affects attitudes toward depression. "Suicide is a very shameful thing in the mountains," said Sammy. "It's considered a sin. You'll go to hell; that's what my family believes." It means you have failed in your faith. It's not your right to "play God" and choose when to die, Sammy said; according to evangelical Christians, it's God's choice. To commit suicide means you renounce God. According to Sammy, people will tell you "to snap out of it. Buck up. Stop crying. Put your feet on the floor and keep going. Toughen up." You need to have stronger faith, and at church, she said, "you would be expected to go to the altar and ask forgiveness for wallowing in your misery, because that's sinful. God is good to you, and you have to count your blessings. Don't worry about things you can't have any control over."

Nobody from her family's Baptist church or the Methodist church she now attends has ever called to offer support in her suffering. "You're an embarrassment," Sammy said. "I wasn't allowed to tell anyone at school after I came back from trying to commit suicide. I wasn't allowed to go to the counselor at school or to tell the principal. I had embarrassed my father because he was a Baptist preacher. He was an evangelist. He did tent meetings, tent revivals, and went to preach at revivals at different churches. I would have ruined any chance of him ever getting a church if it had gotten out that I had done that. He would never have been able to preach again." Without any social support, Sammy suffered a heavy burden after her suicide attempt. "It was just pure isolation," she said, "and shame and guilt."

After her marriage to a local man, Sammy had a baby, and when she suffered from "the baby blues" afterward, her general practitioner put her on an antidepressant, and she began to feel better. However, her husband, Kyle, would not let her get a refill. She remembered that her husband said, "You shouldn't depend on pills." He felt it was a waste of money and that if she simply tried harder, she could pull herself out of it on her own. Kyle has had a long history of alcohol and drug abuse, and Sammy suffered from domestic violence over the course of their marriage. After their divorce, Kyle was arrested for statutory rape of a minor and was put in a psychiatric hospital for two years awaiting trial due to mental incompetence with bipolar disorder. He was in jail at the time of the interview. Kyle's brother committed suicide many years ago, and according to Sammy, Kyle's mother (Sammy's former mother-in-law) "is still struggling over that because she thinks he will be in hell. She thinks you have no chance of going to heaven if you commit suicide." Sammy's daughter is currently being treated for Major Depressive Disorder. Mental illness clearly runs on both sides of the family.

Sammy continues to suffer from bouts of depression. She responds, as she says, by "caving," just going into the bedroom and hiding: "If you're not out working and looking good and contributing to society, then you're shameful, you're an embarrassment." She is a substitute school teacher in an adjacent county, and depression keeps her from working sometimes. She has been to mental health professionals over the years, including a Christian counselor who she thinks was "wonderful." She is on antidepressants and believes the medication is helpful. She also finds writing cathartic, and she loves gardening, hiking, Tai Chi, and dancing in her living room. But she is afraid that the school system will find out that she suffers from depression. Sammy knows a peer support counselor who had a nervous breakdown when she was a teacher, and they fired her. "You just don't do that around here," said Sammy. "I mean if someone has cancer, they do everything in the world to try to help them. But if somebody's got depression, they do not consider it an illness. It's a weakness, not an illness." Sammy has reason to be anxious; she says she was fired by the school system after she married a Mexican man a few years ago and has only been able to get substitute teaching jobs in the county since then.

Scholars in Appalachian Studies would find several manifestations of mountain values in Sammy's words (see Jones 1994). The idea of independence and self-reliance is clearly present in the description of her family's encouragement to stop crying, snap out of it, pick yourself up, and keep going. Also present is the value of hard work and effort and the desire not to look lazy by staying in bed all day. Characterizing depression as a weakness might be interpreted as a general moral weakness in character in someone who refuses to get up and get to work. In other cases in our study, consultants mentioned that it is inappropriate to seek out social attention when sick due to the value of humility and keeping a low profile in the mountains. However, the overriding reference to religious concerns in Sammy's case leads us to consider a different framework for interpreting this weakness that leads to the shameful condemnation of the entire community: it is a spiritual weakness.

Evangelical Christianity and the Cultural Context

A number of questions arise from Sammy's case. What are the cultural beliefs in Appalachian communities that create a context of intense shame involving the experience of depression-like symptoms? Why would a family's shame prevent them from making use of mental health professionals and medications when a family member like Sammy has severe depression, especially when suicide is believed to have such devastating eternal consequences? Why would families, especially those like Sammy's in which severe depression and serious mental disturbances affect many family members, not jump at the chance to control symptoms with medication and other forms of orthodox treatment? What is different about emotional suffering (because there is no similar reticence among native Appalachians to make use of medical services for physical illness)? Why is it difficult for people to even talk about depression in Appalachia—including within families touched by severe forms of the illness? Why should evangelical churches, preachers, and congregation members in rural Appalachia (normally characterized as forming supportive communities) respond to members suffering from depression-like symptoms with avoidance and, sometimes, ostracism?

Most native Appalachians are evangelical Christians; they believe in God and try to develop a personal relationship with God through prayer. The most common evangelical religious affiliations in the mountains are Baptist, Methodist, and Pentecostal-Holiness, and churches in rural areas are typically small and independent of hierarchical associations (such as the Southern Baptist Association). As fundamentalists, evangelical Christians in the mountains agree on the five fundamentals of faith: (1) the infallibility of the Holy Bible, (2) the Virgin Birth, (3) the resurrection of Jesus Christ, (4) Christ's atonement on the cross for the sins of humanity, and (5) the Second Coming when Jesus will return for believers (Riesebrodt 1993, 10). From the evangelical Christian viewpoint, God is in control of all things in heaven and on earth. This includes the emotional life of believers.

Evangelical Christians agree that humans have fallen away from God due to original sin, but this separation from God can be overcome through an emotional heartfelt encounter with the divine. First, sinners must repent and affirm their belief and faith in the Savior, Jesus Christ. Believers are then urged to seek a personal relationship with God once they are "born again."

For Evangelicals, when one is born again, God enters your heart. You surrender your will, give up everything, and welcome God into your heart to work through you. The Holy Spirit "warms" your heart, comes to dwell within you, and you feel joy/bliss/peace/love. This is love in the sense of the Christian religious concept of agape, or charitable, selfless, altruistic, and unconditional love—as God is believed to love humanity. Early evangelical Christian leaders wrote about this feeling. In 1738, John Wesley described in his journal when responding to a speaker who was describing "the change which God works in the heart through faith in Christ, I felt my heart strangely warmed. I felt I did trust in Christ, Christ alone for my salvation" (in Noll 2001, 11). In another example, early-eighteenth-century evangelist Charles Finney, talked about feeling "waves and waves of liquid love" during a religious service (in Luhrmann 2012, 147). Evangelical Christians today speak of being "filled with the Spirit" when the Holy Spirit is working through them, and they often sense the spirit of God flowing through their bodies (something like electricity) as well as filling their hearts. In this new life as an evangelical Christian, God takes control of your life, and your actions as well as your emotions become "God-driven." Your suffering is lifted by Jesus through his suffering on your behalf on the cross. God is said to love and accept you just as you are. Moreover, evangelical Christians believe that humans were created in the image of God for the purpose of enjoying His fellowship, that God wants to be your confidant and wants you to come to Him in prayer (Noll 2001).

The heart is the locus of this change in the new believer. God, in the form of the Holy Spirit, works on the heart. In the Bible, Luke 6:45 (King James Version), Jesus says, "A good man out of the good treasure of his heart bringeth forth that which is good; and an evil man out of the evil treasure of his heart bringeth forth that which is evil: for of the abundance of the heart his mouth speaketh." In other passages, Jesus (Mark 8:17) and the Holy Spirit (Hebrews 3:8) warn against the hardening of hearts to the word of God. Evangelical Christians understand God to be breaking through the "wall of reason" to touch the heart (Mathews 1977, 12). As the heart is moved and transformed by these religious affections, these feelings begin to operate on a higher plane of existence, ultimately making an impression on the soul and infusing the believer with grace (McLoughlin 1978). New believers are encouraged to nurture the God within by developing the heart—stretching it to accept more of God's love.

Evangelical Christians do this through many practices including lifelong individual prayer, keeping prayer journals, individual and group Bible study, hymn singing, and worship in church in communal prayer and communal rituals. Mountain people talk about creating "fellowship" with God, just as they work to create fellowship with the members of their church. Often this occurs through firsthand conversations with Jesus, who becomes like a personal friend. In a fascinating ethnography entitled *When God Talks Back*, anthropologist T. M. Luhrmann describes the way in which new evangelical Christian believers learn to recognize the thoughts in their mind that are not their own but, rather, represent God talking to them. Luhrmann says they learn a "new theory of the mind" that is different from common sense, on the one hand, or psychologists' understanding of the mind, on the other (Luhrmann 2012, 41). In this new theory of the mind, believers learn how to recognize thoughts that are from beyond the natural world, from God. In addition to recognizing God's voice, they also learn to recognize the feelings and sensations in their body that emanate from God.

Emotional calm and stability is the norm in the mountains where people are expected to demonstrate self-control and independence of others in their actions. Strong emotions, on the other hand, are enthusiastically unleashed in church, where spontaneous and heartfelt expression of emotion is considered a sign of connection with God (Dorgan 2006). In church, people are allowed to cry without shame. They might physically feel a sense of bliss in God's presence. Commonly in the past, though perhaps less common today, people in church who were moved by the Holy Spirit would shout, or run, or fall to the ground writhing in ecstasy. This is also described in early writings about the revivals that swept through the mountains during the Great Awakening at the turn of the nineteenth century and in the religious awakenings that followed (Mathews 1977). This primacy of the emotions provokes one scholar to call evangelicalism "the democracy of emotion rather than the hierarchy of the intellect" (Mathews 1977, xvi). God is also believed to work directly through individuals, emotionally inspiring them to preach, among other things; in mountain churches, the preachers are often "called" to preach rather than being trained in seminary for religious leadership. Moreover, their preaching in church typically depends on spontaneous and direct inspiration from God rather than being carefully worked out in written sermons (Jones 1999).

While these positive emotions of joy and bliss and love are signs of spiritual inspiration, negative and inappropriate emotional responses such as anger, hatred, pride, lust, envy, greed, worry, self-absorption, and self-doubt are sins and things of the flesh. For Evangelicals, the Holy life is "a constant and ruthless struggle" against worldly temptations, but one that is worth waging (Mathews 1977, 62). Loyal Jones (1999) makes clear that mountain people typically believe in the Devil as well as in God, and these negative emotions are typically understood by evangelical Christians to be the result of the work of the Devil, who is always trying to draw humanity away from God. To submit to Satan's temptations is to sin; hence, the conclusion that suicide is a sin. To question God's Will and unconditional love is a sin; thus, the warning that worry and self-doubt are sins. In the mind of the evangelical Christian, God does not withdraw, rather you pull away. Instead of withdrawing, believers are admonished to remain strong in their faith, to return to prayer, and to resist the temptation to fall away from God. Jesus is typically the intermediary for the emotional concerns of evangelical Christians; one's sins and concerns are confessed directly to Jesus and, thus, to God. Religious leaders are rarely sought out for confessions, although the intercessory prayers of others are welcomed. If another believer is aware of the suffering of others, he or she typically does not probe further but simply responds by saying, "I'll pray for you." The assumption is that resolution requires the work of the sinner himself or herself, who must go to God in prayer.

Feelings of worthlessness, helplessness, and hopelessness, in other words, may be interpreted by evangelical Christians as due to a lack of spiritual strength. These commonly cited symptoms of depression may *not* be understood by evangelical Christians as a mental health problem requiring the care of a therapist. Instead, appropriate healing would require the individual to pray and to seek God's help. Turning to a mental health professional might not only be seen as inappropriate but misleading, since most mental health professionals use secular therapeutic models that do not specifically incorporate religious healing. Christian counselors, on the other hand, are known to incorporate spirituality and prayer in their understanding and treatment of emotional problems. Several of our cases, including Sammy, spoke highly of the Christian counselors they consulted.

Evangelical Christians do not conceptualize themselves as atomistic individuals with self-contained feelings and emotions triggered by social or environmental factors. Instead, their emotions are interpreted as an outcome of their relationship with God, or the lack thereof. Through faith, God works through them as they endeavor to become "good Christians" and to transcend their sinful nature. Self-scrutiny is the means by which they assess their success in following the path of Jesus Christ. Sinful behavior, often interpreted to include drinking, taking drugs, swearing, fornicating, smoking, or dancing, is to be avoided. Other behavior often believed to be immoral and sinful by evangelical Christians includes homosexuality, premarital sex, abortion, divorce and remarriage, many symptoms of depression (including feeling worthless and hopeless), and forms of outrageous behavior deemed bizarre or "crazy." Individuals are assumed to be responsible for these sinful behaviors and are expected to reform. In addition, church discipline may be used to sanction these kinds of behavior in individual members, who may be called out by name during a sermon in church or made to suffer shunning or ostracism by the congregation (Mathews 1977). However, congregants generally remind themselves to "hate the sin; love the sinner." Thus, religious healing is always possible since God's love is considered to be unconditional. By "making it right with God" through confession, repentance, and the receipt of God's forgiveness in prayer, evangelical Christians believe they can overcome their sins, reform, and find peace.

Evangelical Christians in rural Appalachia often have little understanding of mental illness in the modern psychological sense. In fact, their religious stance rejects a secular, scientific, and naturalistic view of the world. Instead, they see their health and well-being as coming from God. This includes their emotional as well as their physical health. They have come to accept the healing powers of physicians because they see God working through doctors and medications to heal the physical body. In this sense, they have a holistic view of healing. On the other hand, they do not subscribe to Cartesian dualism, which perceives mind and body as separate from one another. Instead, they make a distinction between physical versus spiritual problems, and mental and emotional disturbances are for the most part connected with the spiritual dimension. This distinction becomes clear when considering the folk illness "nerves." Only one of our consultants identified as having nerves, which typically was equated with anxiety and nervousness and not the symptoms of major depression experienced by most of our cases. Our consultants perceived nerves as having somatic symptoms which are appropriately treated by a physician with "nerve pills" such as Xanax or Valium.

Emotional problems are more likely to be understood as in need of spiritual healing. A number of our consultants, like Sammy, describe learning about psychology in high school or college courses, perhaps first identifying depression as a medical diagnosis there. Many have learned extensive psychological language and causal models, likely as a result of years, sometimes decades, of treatment and, often, hospitalization. Most have accepted that they have a chronic illness that requires medication. Many have families that have learned, through the experience of one of their own, about the biopsychosocial model of depression and have become more supportive of mental health treatment. Most have learned various ways of coping with the shame they feel in their community, often resorting to relocation to find anonymity.

Conclusion

In conclusion, the beliefs of evangelical Christianity are at odds with modern medicine and psychology on the derivation of emotions and their consequences. Whereas modern psychology understands emotions as fairly universal and resulting from a mixture of biological, evolutionary, cognitive, and social factors (Kim, Thibodeau, and Jorgensen 2011), evangelical Christians see negative emotional states, such as depression, as evidence of spiritual problems in need of God's guidance. Since the majority of the rural population in Appalachia is evangelical Christian, we suspect that these beliefs dominate the cultural context in most rural communities in Appalachia. They also inform the beliefs of many urban Appalachians, and, considering the fact that more than one-third of the American population is evangelical Christian, they undoubtedly inform the beliefs of many communities throughout the South and in other parts of the United States as well. Since evangelical Christianity dominates the religious landscape in Appalachia, mountain communities with religious diversity may find that even the attitudes and feelings of people of other faiths are affected by these beliefs.

Although, in general, research has found an inverse relationship between religion/spirituality and depression, for a subset of people who may experience themselves as falling short of the expectations of their religion, religion and spirituality appear to be related to greater depression (Bonelli et al. 2012). Specifically, Bonelli and colleagues, in their review of over four hundred studies across the last fifty years that examined the relationship between religious/ spiritual involvement and depression or depressive symptoms, found relatively high levels of depression among those who identified as Pentecostal, although the relationship between the two is unclear and correlational. In addition, they found that involvement in religion/spirituality predicted greater symptoms of depression for those who reported family problems as opposed to other problems such as financial or health problems. The authors hypothesize that those religious beliefs that place great value on family may result in greater guilt, and, in turn, depression. Indeed, Kim and colleagues in their meta-analytic review found that guilt related to an exaggerated sense of responsibility for uncontrollable events, as well as "free-floating" guilt, was associated with depression (Kim, Thibodeau, and Jorgenson 2011).

For evangelical Christians, emotions typically attributed to those suffering from depression, such as feelings of worthlessness, hopelessness, and helplessness, are not immediately recognized as symptoms of mental illness but rather as spiritual problems emanating from humanity's sinful nature. As such, they are stigmatized emotions that people hide from others, including close friends and family (as well as social scientists). To speak of them is to admit sin, and so no language exists to speak about them without condemnation. Evangelicals respond by redoubling their religious practices and socially isolating themselves to avoid public humiliation. For those whose efforts are unsuccessful and whose problems become known due to hospitalization or a suicide attempt, the victim not only experiences individual guilt but also shame and communal sanctions including avoidance and, in some cases, ostracism. For those who commit suicide, they leave behind family members who suffer embarrassment for their inability to lead the victim back to God's fold, grief at the loss of their loved one, and pain in the knowledge that they will never again see their family member who is damned to hell for eternity.

These beliefs have contributed to the growth of Christian counselors in recent decades as evangelical Christians search for culturally appropriate forms of treatment. The American Association of Christian Counselors, for example, has over fifty thousand members and claims as its mission "to equip clinical, pastoral, and lay care-givers with biblical truth and psychosocial insights that minister to hurting persons and helps them move to personal wholeness, interpersonal competence, mental stability, and spiritual maturity" (American Association of Christian Counselors 2014). Three private colleges in North Carolina offer degrees in Christian counseling. For many Evangelicals, Christian counseling is a clear alternative to secular mental health services because it incorporates Christian spiritual practices (including prayer) with psychological counseling, blending the benefits of both. Few Christian counselors practice openly in secular settings such as community mental health centers or state-supported mental hospitals. Perhaps hiring Christian counselors is perceived as a conflict of church versus state or religion versus science. However, given the need for well-trained therapists who can provide culturally competent mental health care in the Appalachian region, mental health agencies would do well to consider better integrating religion and spirituality into public services. Preliminary investigations of actively addressing and utilizing faith in the context of mental health interventions suggest this may be fruitful (Smith, Bartz, and Richards 2007). Furthermore, college-based training programs should actively train practitioners to consider religion and spirituality in the assessment and treatment of depression as well as other forms of emotional suffering. Professional journals such as *Psychology of Religion and Spirituality*, published by the American Psychological Association, are evidence of promise in addressing this gap.

Given the difference between the evangelical Christian-shaped worldview of Appalachian natives and that of modern psychology, we were lucky to get any volunteers in our study at all. Because we solicited volunteers who had experienced depression or took anti-depressants, we largely collected a sample of consultants who had adopted the biopsychosocial model of mental health professionals. Yet, their illness narratives reveal a rich cultural context, complicating our original thinking. Future research on mental health and illness in Appalachia will do well to take religion in general and evangelical Christianity, specifically, into consideration.

---

[1] All names used in the case study are pseudonyms.

Works Cited

Abela J. R., and D. U. D'Alessandro. 2002. "Beck's Cognitive Theory of Depression: A Test of the Diathesis-Stress and Causal Mediation Components." *British Journal of Clinical Psychology* 41:111-28.

American Association of Christian Counselors. 2014. Mission. Accessed July 9. http://www.aacc.net/about-us.

American Psychiatric Association. 2013. Diagnostic and Statistical Manual of Mental Disorders-5. Washington, DC: American Psychiatric Association.

American Psychological Association. 2012. Recognition of Psychotherapy Effectiveness, http://www.apa.org/about/policy/resolution-psychotherapy.aspx.

Antonuccio, D. O., W. G. Danton, and G. Y. DeNelsky. 1995. "Psychotherapy Versus Medication for Depression: Challenging the Conventional Wisdom with Data." *Professional Psychology: Research and Practice* 26:574-85.

Beck, A. T. 1979. *Cognitive Therapy of Depression*. New York: Guilford Press.

Bonelli, R. M., R. E. Dew, H. G. Koenig, R. H. Rosmarin, and S. Vasegh. 2012. "Religious and Spiritual Factors in Depression: Review and Integration of the Research." *Depression Research and Treatment*. doi:10.1155/2012/962860.

Dorgan, Howard. 2006. "Religion." In *Encyclopedia of Appalachia*, edited by Rudy Abrahmson and Jean Haskell. Knoxville: University of Tennessee Press. Section IV, 1281-89.

Engel G. L. 1977. "The Need for a New Medical Model: A Challenge for Biomedicine." *Science* 196:129–36.

Friedman, R. A. 2012. "Perspective: Grief, Depression and the DSM-5." *New England Journal of Medicine* 366:1855-57.

Halverson, J. A., L. Ma, and E. J. Harner. 2004. *An Analysis of Disparities in Health Status and Access to Health Care in the Appalachian Region.* Washington, DC: Appalachian Regional Commission.

Hauenstein, E. J., and S. D. Peddada. 2007. "Prevalence of Major Depressive Episodes in Rural Women Using Primary Care." *Journal of Health Care for the Poor and Underserved* 18:185-202.

Huttlinger, K., J. Schaller-Ayers, and T. Lawson. 2004. "Health Care in Appalachia: A Population-Based Approach." *Public Health Nursing* 21:103-10.

Jones, Loyal. 1994. *Appalachian Values.* Ashland, KY: Jesse Stuart Foundation.

———. 1999. *Faith and Meaning in the Southern Uplands.* Urbana: University of Illinois Press.

Kim, S., R. Thibodeau, and R. S. Jorgenson. 2011. "Shame, Guilt and Depressive Symptoms: A Meta-analytic Review." *Psychological Bulletin* 137: 68-96.

Kleinman, Arthur. 1980. *Patients and Healers in the Context of Culture.* Berkeley: University of California.

Lazarus, R. S. 1993. "From Psychological Stress to the Emotions: A History of Changing Outlooks." *Annual Review of Psychology* 44:1-21.

Luhrmann, T. M. 2012. *When God Talks Back: Understanding the American Evangelical Relationship with God.* New York: Alfred A. Knopf.

Mathews, Donald G. 1977. *Religion in the Old South.* Chicago: University of Chicago Press.

McLoughlin, William G. 1978. *Revivals, Awakenings, and Reform: an Essay on Religion and Social Change in America, 1607-1977*. Chicago: University of Chicago Press.

Muntaner, C., and E. Barnett. 2000. "Depressive Symptoms in Rural West Virginia: Labor Market and Health Services Correlates." *Journal of Health Care for the Poor and Underserved* 11: 284-300.

Noll, Mark A. 2001. *American Evangelical Christianity: an Introduction*. Oxford: Blackwell.

Olfson, M., and S. C. Marcus. 2010. "National Trends in Outpatient Psychotherapy." *American Journal of Psychiatry* 167:1456-63.

Riesebrodt, Martin. 1993. *The Emergence of Modern Fundamentalism in the United States and Iran*. Berkeley: University of California Press.

Saveanu, Ranu, V., and Charles B. Nemeroff. 2012. "Etiology of Depression: Genetic and Environmental Factors." *Psychiatric Clinics of America* 3:51-71.

Smith, T. B., J. Bartz, and P. S. Richards. 2007. "Outcomes of Religious and Spiritual Adaptations to Psychotherapy: A Meta-analytic Review." *Psychotherapy Research* 17(6): 643-55.

World Health Organization. 1992. International Statistical Classification of Diseases and Related Health Problems-10. Geneva: World Health Organization.

Zhang, Z., A. Infante, M. Meit, N. English, M. Dunn, and K. H. Bowers. 2008. *An Analysis of Mental Health and Substance Abuse Disparities and Access to Treatment Services in the Appalachian Region*. Washington, DC: Appalachian Regional Commission.

Idioms of Distress among White Women Patients at the Southwestern Lunatic Asylum, Marion, Virginia, 1887-1891

Anthony P. Cavender

I. Introduction

In 1919, Victor Tausk, a psychoanalyst who studied under Sigmund Freud, wrote a provocative paper, "On the Origin of the 'Influencing Machine' in Schizophrenia," in which he explored the content of his patients' delusions (Tausk 1933). He observed a common pattern in his patients' delusions, one which entailed the manifestation of an "influencing machine" that controlled people's minds and bodies, and he concluded that the imagery they expressed (hidden batteries, radios, magic lanterns, phonographs, dynamos, x-ray machines) reflected the rapid transformation of society. Unlike his mentor, he did not argue that modernity created new forms of mental illness, but that the changing cultural landscape offered patients new symbols to express their diseased mental states.

Studies done over the years on what has come to be termed *idioms of distress* or *languages of distress* elucidate how mentally ill persons unconsciously or consciously draw upon a repertoire of symbols within their culture to express mental disorders. An often cited example in anthropology is Scheper-Hughes' work (1979, 1987) on schizophrenia among the Irish in rural Ireland and those of Irish descent in South Boston. She found that the Irish frequently expressed their illnesses in religious constructs of guilt and persecution and in delusions associated with the Virgin Mary and the Saviour. Her findings align with earlier research done on the differences in idioms of distress used by Irish American compared to Italian American schizophrenics (Singer and Opler 1956). The cultural patterning of idioms of distress has also been examined among women in south India (Nichter 1981), Mexican and Anglo Americans (Weisman et al. 2000), and African Americans (Whaley and Hall 2009). There are perhaps no better examples of culture as a determinant in the expression of mental illness than the numerous cultural syndromes identified worldwide, such as *susto* and *nervios* among Latinos, Japanese disorders like *kitsunetsuki* and *hikkomori,* and *windigo* and *piblotok* among Native North Americans. A commonly held notion is that cultural syndromes are not unique to the culture where they exist; rather, they are labels for a universally shared set of scientifically identifiable mental disorders that manifest in contrasting somatic and symbolic idioms of distress: *susto* is an anxiety disorder, *windigo* is a personality disorder, and so forth. Some research considers how idioms of distress are reflective of and influenced by certain social situations. For example, a rural, undereducated man living in poverty in Southern Appalachia who says, "I've got a bad case of the nerves," is actually saying, "I'm distressed by poverty" (Van Shaik 1988). Susto among Latino migrants in the United States is seen as an inability to cope with an alien world (Dura-Villá and Hodes 2012). More recently, Nichter (1981) advocated for a more expansive and nuanced model for understanding idioms of distress, one that embraces the "micropolitical" context and the polysemic/multivocal dynamics of somatic and symbolic expressions of distress.

Drawing on the underlying assumption of the idiom of distress (i.e., culture is a determinant in the somatic and symbolic presentation of mental illness) as a point of departure, this paper examines the thematic content of the delusions and obsessions expressed by white women patients at the Southwestern Lunatic Asylum in Marion, Virginia, from 1887 to 1891, focusing on how the repertoire of symbols used reflects local and national cultural contexts.

II. The Setting: Southwestern Lunatic Asylum

Southwestern Lunatic Asylum (now the Southwestern Virginia Mental Health Institute, hereafter referred to as "Southwestern") was constructed in 1887 toward the end of the great boom in asylum building in the United States. Its construction was prompted by over-crowding at Eastern Lunatic Asylum in Williamsburg, America's first publicly supported asylum; Western Lunatic Asylum in Staunton; and Pinel Hospital, an institution established to treat people suf-fering from alcohol and drug (i.e., opiates) addiction (Blanton 1933, 206-9). No doubt, Central Lunatic Asylum in Petersburg, established in 1868 expressly for blacks, was overcrowded as well, but patients there could not be transferred to the other white-only institutions.

Southwestern was by any measure of the time a fully modern psy-chiatric facility. Architecturally, it followed the so-called "Kirkbride plan" with a central administration building and two wings attached, one for women and the other for men. It had incandescent light-ing, sophisticated ventilation and fire control systems, innovative kitchens and dining facilities, beautifully groomed landscapes, and a farm worked by the patients that provided much of the food con-sumed by the patients and staff. The medical staff initially included three physicians, all of them well trained. Dr. Robert J. Preston, a native Virginian, served as superintendent of Southwestern from 1887 to 1906. An alienist[1] of national prominence who served as president of the American Medico-Psychological Association (now the American Psychiatric Association) in 1902 (Hurd, Drewry, and Dewey 1916), Preston was a staunch advocate of what was called "moral treatment"[2] even though it was falling out of favor in the psychiatric community in the late nineteenth century (Preston 1887, 1888, 1889).

Patient Sample

The medical records of 461 women admitted to Southwestern from 1887 to 1891 were reviewed for this study (Records of Southwestern State Hospital 1887 to 1948). The women came from all parts of Virginia, though the majority resided in small towns and hamlets in southwestern Virginia, and a few were from out of state. Women of various social classes are represented. The relatively high social status of some women is indicated by their designation as "pay patients," which meant that their family's level of wealth required them to pay for their treatment. A few of the wealthier women brought a servant with them. The medical records are unclear as to how many pay patients there were, but it appears that most of the women met the criteria to qualify for paying no fee. At the other end of the spectrum was what the staff called "the cornfield lady"—that is, the woman associated with the subsistence farming way of life. Occupationally, most of the women were classified as housekeepers and housemaids. Other occupations were seamstress, schoolteacher, cook, and laborer. Several women were identified as having "no occupation" and a few were tagged as "vagrants."

The medical records contain basic demographic information, such as age, marital status, number of children birthed, and residence. Time of onset of insanity is noted along with the symptoms and whether the disorder had "increased" or "decreased" over time. The "form of insanity" was not always recorded in the records. Nevertheless, the forms of insanity and associated number of patients suffering from them appear in the superintendent's annual report to the state. The nosology of insanity includes four types of mania, two types of melancholia, and five types of dementia, toxic insanity, and imbecility.

Prior treatment and asylum occupancy, if any, are noted, as well as the physical condition of the patient. Interest at the time in the heritability of insanity prompted the gathering of information on other family members who currently were or had been insane. The remainder of the record is a description of a patient's behavior during her stay, treatments administered, ward placements, furloughs home, and date and time of discharge. Some patients, most of them older, long-term residents, died while under care. The date, time, and cause of death are noted in these cases.

Information on the subjects of derangement was obtained from the symptomology section of the records. It was commonly expressed as "She is deranged on the subject of . . ." or "Her derangement is evinced on the subject of . . ." The subjects of derangement appear to be associated with an abnormal obsession with a particular topic or a prominent feature of a delusional state. Derangement subjects were not reported for all patients, including epileptics, imbeciles, and those suffering from severe enervation and some physical diseases like tuberculosis and trachoma. As shown in table 1, the majority of the women patients exhibited a generalized form of derangement apparently manifesting in a constantly changing constellation of different subjects. There were, however, subjects that were more fixed and common among several patients, such as, (in descending order of the number of reports): religion[3], property, fear of being harmed or killed, marriage and love, and committing an unpardonable sin. It is important to note that some of the subjects of derangement are idiosyncratic. One patient, for example, claimed that she was the wife of Abraham Lincoln. An accomplished opera singer from Richmond maintained that she had a vine growing up her body from her feet to her eyes and that her husband's head was a skull. Another woman claimed that a table she had recently purchased was "haunted" and caused her and her family great misfortune.

Subject of Derangement	Reports	Percentage
General	81	28.4
Religion	62	21.7
Property	37	12.9
Fear of Harm	29	10.1
Marriage/Love	16	5.6
Unpardonable Sin	10	3.5
Death	8	2.8
Jealousy of Husband	8	2.8
Abandonment by Husband	5	1.7
Witchcraft	5	1.7
Cluverius	4	1.4
Freemasonry	4	1.4
Harm to Children	4	1.4
Nymphomania	4	1.4
Devil	3	1.0
Fire	3	1.0
Cleanliness	1	>1.0
Spiritualism	1	>1.0
TOTAL	285	100

Table 1. Subjects of Derangement Reported by Patients

Space limitations preclude an analysis of all the subjects of derangement presented in table 1. Five subjects, therefore, are chosen, including the two most frequently reported, religion and property, and, to demonstrate periodicity, three less frequently reported, "Negroes," Freemasonry, and the famous trial of Thomas J. Cluverius.

Religion

Importantly, religious insanity or, as it was alternately called, "religious excitement" or "religious mania," was not solely an expression of insanity; it was also seen as a discrete form and cause of insanity. Equally important, religious insanity was not a uniquely southern phenomenon. The origin of the disorder in America goes back to the

First Great Awakening in the early 1700s in Pennsylvania and New Jersey, and later to the Second Great Awakening of the early 1800s, which spread from the North to the southern states of Tennessee, Kentucky, and North Carolina. Following the lead of highly esteemed alienists like Amariah Brigham and Pliny Earle, by the mid-1800s, it was widely accepted that the fire and brimstone preaching and the ecstatic experiences induced by revivals, camp meetings, and prolonged church services caused insanity, as did protracted discussions of religious subjects and solitary reading and meditation on the Bible (Bainbridge 1984). Brigham (1835, 285) believed that women were more susceptible to religious insanity than men because of their more delicate nervous systems, but national statistics do not support his assertion (Bainbridge 1984, 228), nor do the statistics at Southwestern (Preston 1887, 1888, 1889, 1890, 1891) where religious excitement was assigned as the cause of insanity only slightly more among women.

Derangement on the subject of religion involved several obsessive behaviors, most commonly praying aloud, shouting praises, repetitious recitation of scriptures, singing hymns, preaching to others, and reading the Bible. These behaviors were considered normal in some church and revival settings, but if performed incessantly in the home or secular public settings, then one was deemed insane. As for delusional behaviors, one patient maintained that she was a saint and another claimed to be able to communicate with God through her feet. Item 6 in table 1, "Commitment of Unpardonable Sin," and item 16, "The Devil," could reasonably be considered as subsets of the religion category since both are derivatives of the Christian belief system. The following three cases illustrate religion both as a cause and as an expression of insanity.

Ann Drewry, a resident of Petersburg, age 38, married with four children, was described upon admission as incoherent, engaging in excessive talking, nervous, and suffering insomnia. After a few days, it was noted that she "seemingly has no mind at all, feeble, looks stupid and dazed." The cause of her insanity was listed as "Hard and constant study of the Bible."

Julia Felts, a resident of Wise County, age 25, widow with three children, is described as "a woman of temperate habits" who displayed a "gloomy disposition" and was "absent minded." She was for the most part "orderly and quiet," but manifested "much enthusiasm on religious subjects." The cause of her insanity was "grief from the death of her husband who was shot down at her home and in her presence by a drunken mob."

Minnie Tanner of Lynchburg, age 21, unmarried schoolteacher, was admitted suffering from "brain fever" caused by excessive study for examinations. She displayed symptoms of partial paralysis, feebleness, and nervous exhaustion. "Her derangement," it is noted, "is evinced on the subject of religion."

The notion that people in the South in the 1880s would resort to religious symbols and behaviors as an idiom of distress should not surprise us. Historically, southerners are well known for their reliance on religion to psychologically cope with the misfortunes of life. More interesting is the flow of religious symbols and behaviors into the nation's "symptom pool." As defined by medical historian Edward Shorter, a "symptom pool" is a set of patterned symptoms cooperatively identified by both laypeople and physicians as legitimate expressions of mental illness. The symptom pool, Shorter observes, changes over time; mental illnesses regularly appear and disappear. Once commonly diagnosed mental illnesses in nineteenth-century America like hysteria, neurasthenia, puerperal fever, and nymphomania morphed into other forms or vanished altogether. Religious insanity as an official mental disorder also vanished in the early twentieth century (Bainbridge 1984, 236).

Property

Like religion, property was both an idiom and cause of insanity. As used in the medical records, the term *property* seems to refer mainly to house and land, but occasionally there is mention of cash savings. The most frequently reported language of obsession in this category was "fear of want" or "fear of coming to want," meaning a fear of slipping into poverty, similarly expressed as an obsessive fear of being sent to the poorhouse. Contextual information is lacking in the records, but in cases involving subsistence farming families, one can imagine a relatively quick plunge into destitution caused by crop failure, sickness, physical disability, or the loss of livestock, especially a plow animal. As for the impact of sickness on the local economy, the medical records show the presence in the patient population of several diseases that are severely debilitating and potentially fatal, such as malaria, "flux" (dysentery), typhoid, tuberculosis, scrofula, trachoma, erysipelas, pellagra, pneumonia, and influenza. In some cases, a fall into destitution or fear of destitution was prompted by a woman's husband abandoning her and her children. Of relevance to this discussion is that in many instances the medical records state that "she has no property of her own" or that "her husband has property worth . . . ," which indicates that though women at the time had the legal right to own property, many did not.

The many safety nets in the form of government assistance programs taken for granted in America today did not exist in the late nineteenth century. One depended upon kith and kin to get through hard times, but there were limitations to the assistance they could provide. Churches and religious agencies offered limited relief, if they offered any at all. Watkinson (2000, 18) maintains that during the antebellum period in Virginia ministers were more concerned about spiritual poverty than temporal poverty and that churches "gave little aid to the indigent, especially in rural areas, either for doctrinal reasons or due their own straitened circumstances." Many rural counties could not afford to support a poorhouse; thus, many poor people became vagrants and wandered from place to place seeking comfort and not a few of them were placed in jails. This situation persisted in rural Appalachia until the turn of the twentieth century when major denominations like the Presbyterians, Methodists, and Congregationalists became more oriented toward temporal poverty and established settlement schools and installed various economic relief programs in the region (Shapiro 1978). The following four cases illustrate how property figured into an idiom of distress:

Theresa Lauthern, age 47, of Smyth County, a widow with two children, was one of the first patients admitted to Southwestern. Described as a "small, laboring woman," she had first been sent to the county jail for attempting violence to others. Diagnosed with "acute mania," her record states that her insanity was caused by living in poverty. She was discharged "as fully restored to sanity" after six months. She was readmitted, however, less than a month later "after she found her home torn up, household property sold, and her children in the poor house—that all the neighbors treated her badly and almost drove her from the community."

Amanda Albert, age unknown, of Pulaski County, was in a dire situation. She had given birth to seven children in twelve years, and her husband had recently died. Her record states that "she has been overworked and overtaxed—is very poor." She was diagnosed as suffering from neurasthenia (a nervous condition).

Sarah Tinsley, age 55, of Bland County, became insane around the age of 40 due to a loss of property, social status, and beauty. The circumstances attending her family's transition from a life of comfortable affluence to indigence is not indicated. She lived in a delusional world of pretending that nothing had really changed: "She was once a beautiful woman, but since her change in position in life and the loss of beauty, she has occupied herself chiefly at the table with looking glass, paints, and hair brush in hand, primping and trying to resuscitate her lost beauty."

Another dimension of property as a subject of derangement is evident in the delusion of possessing great wealth, often as a claim of owning large tracts of land. Alice Lewis, age 28, of Lynchburg, married with two children, maintained that she had great wealth and owned large tracts of land in Florida "which she thinks someone is trying to rob her of." False claims of ownership of large tracts of land in Florida and California were mentioned by two other patients.

Fear and Hatred of Negroes

The Fear of Harm category in table 1 is most frequently represented by the belief that one has been harmed, or is going to be harmed, by someone in the family or a member or members of the community, usually in terms of being poisoned or bewitched. The five reports of a fear of being harmed by "negroes" and a hatred of them reveals the predominantly racist attitude of whites at the time.

Prior to but especially after the abolition of slavery in 1865, many white southerners lived in fear that blacks would rise up and seek vengeance for their dehumanizing treatment and, furthermore, that they would seize the property of whites and assume power over them. This fear proved to be unwarranted, but many white southerners obsessed about it.

The medical record for Louisa Turner, age 60, of Richmond, reports: "She is in a melancholy state all the time. Thinks the servants put poison in her food and also make different noises to frighten her and that negroes in general are always trying to take her life."

Queen May Bernard, age 55, "Imagines she sees negroes, out the window, who are going to kill her."

Lucy Purdue, age 28, Bland County "thinks the household will be governed by negroes, and that her dresses and other wearing apparel has been given her by a low class of people and that she will no longer wear them."

Ms. Sanders, age 30, Buckingham County, was deranged "on several subjects, but chiefly hatred of negroes, marriage, and to wander." Her record notes that "when she meets the colored driver, or any other colored person, she gives vent to the most profane and often vulgar language, seeming to get into a violent rage."

Freemasonry

Beginning in the late nineteenth century and continuing to the present, conspiracy theorists have maintained that Freemasonry is a sinister, shadowy organization. Some see it as a religious cult with a plan of salvation that differs from that of the Christian Church. Others believe that it is satanically oriented. More common today is the belief that Freemasons control the world and intend to establish, in the words of some conspiracy theorists, a "New World Order." No doubt, the secrecy attending Freemasonry rituals and its cryptic symbols fueled the public's suspicious imagination (Firestone 2013), as did the fact that many of its members have been prominent Americans, including several presidents and leaders in industry. Four women at Southwestern were deranged on the subject of Freemasonry, but no information is provided in the medical records on exactly what concerned them about the organization.

The Trial of Thomas J. Cluverius

Thomas J. Cluverius was an up-and-coming Richmond lawyer who was hanged on January 24, 1887, for the murder of his cousin, Lillian Madison. While engaged to another woman, Cluverius had an affair with his cousin, and she became pregnant. Seeing no way out of an uncompromising situation, he murdered her (and his child) with a blow to her head and disposed of her body in the city reservoir. The Cluverius trial was what we today would call a "celebrity trial," comparable to the sensational trials of O. J. Simpson, Phil Spector, and Casey Anthony. The *New York Times* covered the trial daily. The citizens of Richmond were enthralled and divided by the trial; some thought he was guilty of murder while others claimed Lillian Madison committed suicide. Cluverius was found guilty and hanged publicly. He maintained his innocence to the end. The city's obsession with the trial prompted a prominent judge to write an editorial for a local newspaper in which he encouraged the public to free themselves of the obsession lest there be bad consequences (Trotti 2008). The medical records are unclear, but it is likely that the women deranged on the subject of Cluverius believed he was innocent with the exception, interestingly, of Lucy Madison, the aunt of Lillian Madison. Admitted six months after the hanging of Cluverius, Lucy had become "random in talk and vague in mind, and emaciated from refusing to eat." Her medical records state: "Her niece, Lillian Madison, having been murdered, she imagines that she has caused the trouble by her talk."

III. Conclusion

The idioms of distress evident among women patients at Southwestern Lunatic Asylum from 1887 to 1891 demonstrate how culture (locally and nationally) serves as a determinant in the expression of mental illness and, furthermore, how the symptom pool of the country changes over time. With respect to the idiom of property, the manifestation of an ostensibly irrational mind in terms of being excitably and obsessively fixed on a concern with property appears to be a rational response to a genuine fear of being or becoming destitute.

The idiom of property also points to the fact that many women were marginalized economically; few of them had property and thus were powerless to control the welfare of themselves and their children. No doubt, the hardscrabble existence of the so-called "cornfield woman" and the birthing and care of several children added additional stress. This fact was not lost upon the medical staff at Southwestern. "Overwork" and "birthing many children in rapid succession" are cited in the medical records as causes of insanity.

The religious idiom was very much part of the national symptom pool at the time. As noted earlier, the national symptom pool is constructed by both laypeople and professionals; sometimes it actually originates among laypeople and is then later endorsed by official medicine. In his study of religious insanity, Bainbridge (1984, 235) states that identifications of religious insanity "were usually made first by family and friends of the afflicted, with doctors often merely accepting these lay diagnoses. Thus, the ideology of religious insanity was part of national culture, accepted by ordinary members of the community, as well as by national opinion leaders."

Derangement on the subject of fear and hatred of Negroes reveals a deeply rooted racism long associated with the South, but also a sense of guilt over the mistreatment and disenfranchisement of blacks. It would be interesting to compare the subjects of derangement of blacks in the medical records of Virginia's asylum for blacks, Central State. How did whites figure into the idioms of distress of blacks?

Derangement on the subjects of Freemasonry and Cluverius illustrate how popular culture tropes were accessed to express mental disorders as well as the temporality of idioms of distress. Freemasonry's association with various conspiracy theories oriented around the subversion of the Christian establishment and democratic ideals lent itself to a paranoid state of mind whereas the Cluverius case aligned well with feelings of persecution and guilt.

Other than showing that idioms of distress are culturally constructed and historically specific, these examples remind us of the importance of the context and contours of idiom expression in discriminating the sane from the insane. They also raise questions relevant to the debate among historians, sociologists, and anthropologists about southern distinctiveness. Was, as McCandless (1996, 4) asks, the South psychiatrically unique in comparison with other regions in the United States? Race has long been identified as a unique feature of southern culture, but race was only marginally expressed as a subject of derangement at Southwestern. The fact that a fear and hatred of Negroes was not a more common idiom of distress, however, does not warrant the conclusion that racism was uncommon in Virginia. Virginia's and the South's lurid history of racism speaks for itself, and racism was and remains a national concern. Compared with data from asylums in the North gathered by Bainbridge (1984, 225), it seems that religious excitement was far more common at Southwestern. His data, however, representing the 1860s and earlier, do not align chronologically. Nevertheless, the Southwestern data shows that religion was a significant aspect of life in the South. As for derangement on the subject of property, it is doubtful that insane women in Virginia were unique in this respect. The disenfranchisement of women was a national problem.

Notes

1. The word *alienist* (from the French *aliéniste*) is an archaic term for a physician who specializes in the treatment of mental illness; also used in reference to someone recognized as a legal authority on insanity.

2. Moral treatment emerged in the late eighteenth and early nineteenth centuries from the work of Philipe Pinel in France and William Tuke in England. The term is a translation of Pinel's *traitment moral*, which referred to a therapeutic approach that focused on interventions designed to treat the mind rather than the body. Pinel advocated releasing patients from chains and allowing them to roam freely on the asylum grounds. He abandoned the use of corporal punishment and harsh medical interventions like bleeding, purging, and blistering. Tuke independently developed a remarkably similar program at the York Retreat in Yorkshire. Pinel and Tuke also agreed that patients, while being treated with respect, must be taught self-control and self-restraint in a caring yet strongly controlled community.

3. As suggested later in the paper, if we combine the "Unpardonable Sin" and "Devil" categories with religion, then religion represents 26.3 percent of the idioms of distress.

Works Cited

Bainbridge, William Sims. 1984. "Religious Insanity in America: The Official Nineteenth-Century Theory." *Sociological Analysis* 45:223-40.

Blanton, Wyndam. 1933. *Medicine in Virginia in the Nineteenth Century*. Richmond: Garrett and Massie.

Brigham, Amariah. 1835. *Observations on the Influence of Religion upon the Health and Physical Welfare of Mankind*. Boston: Marsh, Capon and Lyon.

Dura-Villá, Glòria, and Matthew Hodes. 2012. "Cross-Cultural Study of Idioms of Distress among Spanish Nationals and Hispanic American Migrants." *Social Psychiatry and Psychiatric Epidemiology* 47:1627-37.

Firestone, Roger. 2013. Difficult Questions about Freemasonry. Accessed March 15. http://web.mit.edu/dryfoo/Masonry/Questions/difficult.html.

Hurd, Henry Mills, William Drewry, and Richard Dewey. 1916. *The Institutional Care of the Insane in the United States and Canada*. Baltimore: Johns Hopkins Press.

McCandless, Peter. 1996. *Moonlight, Magnolias, and Madness: Insanity in South Carolina from the Colonial Period to the Progressive Era*. Chapel Hill: University of North Carolina Press.

Nichter, Mark. 1981. "Idioms of Distress: Alternatives in the Expression of Psychosocial Distress." *Culture, Medicine, and Psychiatry* 5:379-408.

_____. 2010. "Idioms of Distress Revisited." *Culture, Medicine, and Psychiatry* 34:401-16.

Preston, Robert J. 1887. *Annual Report of the Southwestern Lunatic Asylum of Marion, Virginia*. Richmond: Wm. Ellis Jones Book and Job Printer.

_____. 1888. *Annual Report of the Southwestern Lunatic Asylum of Marion, Virginia*. Richmond: J. H. O'Bannon, Superintendent of Public Printing.

_____. 1889. *Annual Report of the Southwestern Lunatic Asylum of Marion, Virginia*. Richmond: J. L. Hill Printing Company.

_____. 1890. *Annual Report of the Southwestern Lunatic Asylum of Marion, Virginia*. Richmond: J. H. O'Bannon, Superintendent of Public Printing.

_____. 1891. *Annual Report of the Southwestern Lunatic Asylum of Marion, Virginia*. Richmond: J. H. O'Bannon, Superintendent of Public Printing.

Records of Southwestern State Hospital. 1887 to 1948. Series VI, Patient Records, Female, Number 1, 1887-1890, Number 2, 1889-1891. Richmond: Library of Virginia.

Scheper-Hughes, Nancy. 1979. *Saints, Scholars, and Schizophrenia: Mental Illness in Rural Ireland*. Berkeley: University of California Press.

_____. 1987. "'Mental' in 'Southie': Individual, Family, and Community Responses to Psychosis in South Boston." *Culture, Medicine, and Psychiatry* 11:53-78.

Shapiro, Henry D. 1986. *Appalachia on Our Mind*. Chapel Hill: University of North Carolina Press.

Shorter, Edward. 1992. *From Paralysis to Fatigue*. New York: Free Press.

Singer, Jerome, and Morris Opler. 1956. "Contrasting Patterns of Fantasy and Motility in Irish and Italian Schizophrenics." *Journal of Abnormal and Social Psychology* 53:42-47.

Tausk, Victor. 1933. "On the Origin of the Influencing Machine in Schizophrenia." *Psyhcoanalytic Quarterly* 2:519-56.

Trotti, Michael Ayers. 2008. *The Body in the Reservoir: Murder and Sensationalism in the South*. Chapel Hill: University of North Carolina Press.

Van Schaik, Ellen. 1988. "The Social Context of 'Nerves' in Eastern Kentucky." In *Appalachian Mental Illness*, edited by Susan Keefe, 81-100. Lexington: University of Kentucky Press.

Watkinson, James D. 2000. "Rogues, Vagabonds, and Fit Objects: The Treatment of the Poor in Antebellum Virginia." *Virginia Cavalcade* 49:16-29.

Weisman, Amy G., Steven R. López, Joseph Ventura, Keith H. Neuchterlein, Michael J. Goldstein, and Sun Hwang. 2000. "A Comparison of Psychiatric Symptoms between Anglo-Americans and Mexican Americans with Schizophrenia." *Schizophrenia Bulletin* 26:817-24.

Whaley, Arthur L., and Brittany N. Hall. 2009. "Cultural Themes in the Psychotic Symptoms of African American Psychiatric Patients." *Professional Psychology: Research and Practice* 40:75-80.

Water and Cherokee Healing

Lisa J. Lefler

There are no unsacred places; there are only sacred places and desecrated places.
—Wendell Berry, *Given*

Introduction

One of the many rewards of working with indigenous populations is getting to experience a cultural and historical worldview much different from my own. Even though I grew up near many Cherokee people in our rural, mountainous, biologically diverse region, my language and European heritage did not allow me the same understanding of the world around me. There is much of my culture and history that is shared with that of the Cherokee people, but the bottom line is that I grew up white and an English speaker. My Cherokee friends and peers had a great advantage over me in understanding this beautiful, rich, and ecologically unique place, with thousands of years of experience and adaptation to inform them. Their language and culture allowed them the knowledge of being a part *of* that place, not just *from* that place. In this chapter, I hope that we find a common ground where those of us from the colonizing dominant culture will reflect on one of our most common natural elements—water—and will take away a more "Native science" or indigenous perspective of that which is a part of us and part of everything around us. As physicist David Bohm wrote, "The generic thought processes of humanity incline toward perceiving the world in a fragmentary way, breaking things up which are not really separate (1996, xvi-xvii)."

Recognizing the importance of water to all people in all places, the United Nations declared the beginning of The Decade of Water in 2005. Water is vital and many have said even more important than food. Experts say that about three days is the maximum one can survive without it (Binns 2012). Accessible, potable, and sufficient water is of increasing concern worldwide as issues of climate change, development, and population growth continue to be important. Water has always been understood as an element as essential to survival as air. Even more intimately, at the atomic level we are water. The Colorado Water Information website states that "the human body is more than 60 percent water. Blood is 92 percent water, the brain and muscles are 75 percent water, and bones are about 22 percent water" (2013). The Free Drinking Water website notes that "the human brain is made up of 95 percent water, blood is 82 percent and lungs 90 percent" (2013). We know how important water is for our survival, but this paper will look at how water is part of us physically, culturally, and even spiritually. Water not only represents life and sustainability of life, but is an element universally symbolizing renewal and cleansing. The Eastern Band of Cherokee Indians has long understood water's importance and has provided many mechanisms culturally to exemplify water's sacredness.

For the mountains of Southern Appalachia, water is the essence of life for *all* that live there. A temperate rain forest, this region relies on vast systems of branches, creeks, streams, and rivers that channel mountain valleys and hollows. They are places of residence for mystical creatures, which the Cherokee, who have lived in the region for more than ten thousand years, have described in their oral histories and stories.

However, only in the last two or three decades have inhabitants of this region, both Cherokee and nonnative, become increasingly concerned about the availability of water. They are concerned about water quantity and quality and the properties culturally and historically associated with it and that water be accessible to them for both the mundane and sacred activities in which it has heretofore been used.

As a person of Appalachia, my mother reminded us often that the most sacred of places were mountaintops and where water flowed. To her, these were places to be close to God and close to the best evidence of the beauty of his creation. We would sit in streams, turning over rocks for larvae that made their houses under them. We would seek out turtles and salamanders and crawdads and dam up the creeks to play in. We would fish for food and for pleasure and would seek out the waterfalls and rivers to "be still," and watch, and meditate. People who grew up here relied upon the land and water, not only for a living, but for much more. We relied upon the water for a familiarity of place and a reassurance that our lush, green mountains would always be here.

The Cherokee, the longest continuous inhabitants of this region, explain that their emergence into this world came from a place called Kituwah, which rests along the Tuckasegee River. It is considered *the* Mothertown and is a place of tradition and ceremony. On the Harvard University Pluralism website, Cherokee elder Tom Belt refers to it as one would the Vatican, as "the holy of holies" (2013). It is no accident that Kituwah is a river town. It is nestled in a valley where seven mountaintops can be identified surrounding her, and the river flows to and from this town, reaching out to a myriad of other Cherokee towns, carrying people and products.

The Pluralism Report from Harvard University states:

> One of the most sacred aspects of the Kituwah site is its proximity to the Tuckasegee river. Early Cherokee people settled there because water has always been a very important part of the Cherokee worldview. "The water is a living breathing thing. It has life, has spirit, and we

honor him," Dan Taylor, a representative of the Cherokee Museum, said. He elaborated: "The Cherokee were baptists before there were any Baptists," in reference to a ceremonial purification in which every child took part, shortly after birth. The river's ceremonial significance was also reserved for the end of life, when people would gather there for funeral prayer, and where, according to some accounts, the priest was able to tell whether the death was caused by witchcraft. It is likely that the placement of Kituwah mound was determined by the river, because where it stands the river bends and forks. This forking was crucial for early Cherokee, who used one side of the river for bathing and ceremony, and the other for drinking. (2013)

The Cherokee homeland is a land marbled by water. The Oconaluftee River flows down the mountain some five thousand feet and meets with the Tuckasegee River. People identify where they live by names like Bunches Creek, Adams Creek, Goose Creek, Soco Creek, Fisher Branch, and farther out in tribal lands of Graham County, Snowbird Creek and Buffalo Creek. Across the mountains in Macon County, the ancient mounds of Nikwasi and Cowee are bordered by the Little Tennessee River and upriver, the Cullasaja. Other regional rivers reflect the legacy of Cherokee culture by names such as Chatooga, Cheoa, Hiawassie, Nantahala, and Nolichucky. It is no wonder, then, that water would be an element not only important but central to the belief and healing systems of the Cherokee.

Cherokee Healing Rituals

Historically, most Cherokees built their houses close to water, easily accessing water for reasons from maintaining hygiene to conducting ceremony. Most who have lived among or studied Cherokees quickly recognize the phrase "going to water." This ritual has been associated with traditional Cherokee practices since at least ethnographer James Mooney's research at the turn of the twentieth century.

In "Notebook of a Cherokee Shaman," by Cherokee anthropologists Jack Frederick and Anna Gritts Kilpatrick (1970, 105-6), rivers where Cherokees would go to water were referred to as "the long person." Rivers were imbued with spirit, medicine, and longevity. The website of the Cherokee Nation refers to this as "the Long Man." It states, "The river, or 'Long Man,' was always believed to be sacred, and the practice of going to water for purification and other ceremonies was at one time very common. Today the river or any other body of moving water, such as a creek, is considered a sacred site and going to water is still a respected practice by some Cherokees (2012)."

The Kilpatricks point out that "the 'going to the water' ritual may contain details and procedures that reflect the 'personal preferences of the medicine man' and would be precipitated by particular needs of the client" (1970, 93).

As most healing rituals of the Cherokees involve participation of the client, the ritual reflects principles of reciprocity and an exchange of communication between the medicine person and the person in need of assistance. This dynamic of partnership and the quality of relationship can bear greatly upon the outcome of their work. Unlike expectations of Western medicine to do what the doctor tells you or just take a pill and get better quickly, the Cherokee process of healing involves dual participation and expectation to heal from within and an expected length of time for healing to take place. It involves inclusion of natural resources and the spirit of those resources to make one well.

The Kilpatricks continue to discuss "going to the water" and provide a brief ritual: "The client traditionally stands at dawn at the verge of running water, facing east. The medicine man, standing directly behind his client, states the latter's name and clan and then in a low voice recites the text, after which the client stoops and laves his hands and face. This procedure is enacted four times. The entire ceremony is performed upon four consecutive mornings" (1970).

Again, these are rituals of process, context, and precise language use. Water is both a vehicle of medicine and of spirit. It is also part of the larger context in which medicine is administered. Depending on the purpose, where water is gathered is important. A specific place meant for a type of medicine or in a place that lies in a particular geographic spot where water is gathered can be essential. When to gather water can refer to everything from time of day to time of year or season. The reasons why, where, and when water is collected are determined by the medicine person.

Anthropologist Ray Fogelson mentions in his reference to Eastern Cherokee ceremonies, "In the fall three additional ceremonies were observed. The First Great Moon in mid-October was a medicine dance. It was believed that falling leaves infused local streams and rivers with healing power. Local community members under the supervision of a medicine man would immerse themselves in the curative and protective waters. Medicine men bathed privately to renew their strength for the following year" (2004, 349). Sometimes a specific place along a river would be designated by a sign (i.e., a petroglyph) showing where medicine water should be collected.

According to *The Payne-Butrick Papers* of the early to mid-nineteenth century, "the ground on the banks of rivers and on the shore was more holy than that back from the water. The Indians always had their houses of worship, council houses and ceremonies near water. But the ground under the water was still more sacred than that on the shore" (Anderson, Brown, and Rogers 2010, 237).

The Payne-Butrick Papers also record the importance of water in dreams. "In case someone in a family is sick, and some other member in the family dreams of a stream of low, clear water, the one sick is sure to recover, but if the stream is rising and full, either the sick person or someone else is soon to be very sick." The papers also note, "To dream of seeing water rising round a house is a sign of sickness, but if it falls away without running into the house none will die; but if some of the water runs in, one or more will soon die" (Anderson, Brown, and Rogers 2010, 1-3:238-39).

Several early ethnographers write of water ceremonies conducted for a variety of reasons that may not directly involve one's health, such as ensuring a good hunt, catching fish, or even catching a woman. For example, *The Payne-Butrick Papers* state, "During a hunting expedition all hunters must bathe, plunging seven times every new moon (Nutsawi)" (Anderson, Brown, and Rogers 2010, 1-3, 234-35). The papers go on to record medicines that must be applied and drunk, sweat houses used, plunging into the water, and times of morning and evening when these events take place.

Moravian Records

According to the Moravians during their interactions with Cherokees at Springplace Mission, they observed that "many Cherokees and other Native peoples clung to the traditional ways of traveling the waterways. The Conasauga River and its extensive tributary system supported heavy canoe travel, and many Cherokees came to the Springplace Mission in Canoes. Almost all Cherokee visitors lived in riverine communities and their historical waterway arteries provided the means for communication. The Cherokee landscape teemed with traces of artifacts of bygone peoples that had paddled the same streams centuries ago" (McClinton 2007, 1:24).

In their record, they also mention, "The Cherokees used the nearby limestone springs from the Conasauga River for purification rites before and after the ball play" (McClinton 2007, 1:24). This purification rite continues today and is discussed in more detail in Raymond D. Fogelson's dissertation on Cherokee stickball (1962).

Water was to be understood and treated properly as part of the world order. McClinton explains in her work with the Moravian records, "This World," where the Cherokees lived, existed somewhere "between perfect order and complete chaos." Order and predictability reigned in the "Upper World," and disorder and change characterized the "Under World." The Cherokees tried to keep things associated with opposing sections of the cosmic order separate to avoid dire consequences. For example, the Cherokees used dirt to put out fires, not water. Dirt was from This World, fire was from the Upper World, and water was from the Under World. To mix Upper World and Under World—fire and water—meant pollution, and pollution meant chaos; consequently This World had to mediate by providing dirt to extinguish fire." (McClinton 2007, 1:27)

"The Cherokees' categorization of the cosmos and their desire to keep their classifications pure produced an elaborate ritual and ceremonial system. The Cherokees valued order and believed things should stay in their place; therefore, they attached special meanings to anomalies because these occurred along the interstices of their categorical systems. Substances that belonged inside the body but were expelled received particular attention, and thus breath, blood, and saliva possessed mystical properties that healed or induced death" (McClinton 2007, 1:27).

Other intersections of this and the otherworld can occur at "portals." These are openings that allow one to stand at the cusp of the otherworld, usually *not* something recommended or desired. One such caution will come from elders who advise not to stand or go behind waterfalls as these are considered areas of such portals. There are also portals in rivers and streams, as Cherokee scholar Brett Riggs and Cherokee cultural resource officer T. J. Holland have shared by personal correspondence (2013). The spirit world of water reflected in many petroglyphs along rivers and streams throughout Cherokee country depicts water beings as important cultural icons with meaning and value within Cherokee cosmology, their legacy etched in stone.

The importance of these entities and locations live on in ritual. In Ray Fogelson's article on Cherokee Medico-Magical Beliefs, he speaks to the issues of how those Cherokees who have been influenced or converted to Christianity consider water ceremony and symbolism.

> According to one informant: "When I conjure, I go by the word of God . . . In ceremonies, I use the name of the Lord. When somebody's sick, you take him to the creek, wash his face by dipping with your hand, and wet his breast by the heart. It's like the spirit gives strength, like Baptism. He can feel it. If somebody's lost, it's up to the Creator to point the way. Sort of like prayer. If it wasn't in the power of the Creator, you couldn't make anything move. . . ." Here the ancient Cherokee rite of "going to the water" is neatly reconciled with Christianity. (1961, 220)

Ray's colleague, Cherokee anthropologist Robert K. Thomas, explained Cherokee values and worldview in his article of 1958:

> In a nutshell, the Cherokee world is an ordered system. The system has parts and there are reciprocal obligations between the parts. Cherokees are a "part" and have these kinds of obligations. They have an obligation to maintain harmonious interpersonal relations and if this is done, the system works and everyone has the good life or, just another way, the supernatural is obligated to do its part. . . . This system works in relation between each man and

the universe. Each person's "good life" gets some kind of reward. This theory is the basis of an old Cherokee medical practice. Sickness was brought about because the individual had come into conflict with something in the human, animal, or supernatural world. Then disease is brought by a person working against you, an animal ghost that you have offended or some supernatural force because a taboo has been broken. The cure is brought about by using some technique from the Cherokee store of "knowledge" to combat the sickness. Cherokee medicine can also be used positively to keep interpersonal relations harmonious and to bring one "luck." (22)

In the last several years, I have had the privilege of working with many speakers, women, and elders who are working to revitalize not only language but also ritual and protocols that were in place for the health of their women and children. In these discussions, I am reminded of the connection between our voice, attitudes, energy, and perspectives of our place in this world to health and well-being.

In talking about the importance of finding a place to be calm and thoughtful, an elder in the Snowbird community shared, "One of our enrolled members had Lupus and when she felt really bad, she would go to a rock in the river where she would sit. It calmed her and made her feel better." Another woman said, "There are places along Snowbird Creek where there are trees that sit along the creek bank and those are good places to sit and 'feel better.'"

Western science has not completely ignored the health benefits of providing patients the ability to be close to nature as part of recovery. It has just taken many years of empirical evidence and categorization of types and factors in using landscape therapeutically to catch up with indigenous knowledge about the healing power of nature. Even Florence Nightingale wrote in her *Notes on Nursing* (1860) that the

accessibility of patients to see and connect with the beauty and won-
ders of nature were cathartic. She recommended placing patients
within eyeshot of flowers or natural beauty to aid in their recovery.
Studies since then have encouraging results in what is now called
"landscape therapy." For more thorough references see Shan Jiang's
article "Therapeutic Landscapes and Healing Gardens" (2014).

Related to these discussions, I asked Tom Belt, a friend and colleague who works with the Cherokee language program and elders,
about his understanding of "getting well" and whether there is a connection to place. He replied, "We are related to all things as all things
are related to each other. These are very real connections. Change of
cycles, moon, and other natural elements were all things that needed
to be noticed, just as human existence also is looked at in a cyclic
way. We all change physically, emotionally, and spiritually. There is
an 'order' to things and things happen in ways they are supposed to
that we can't tamper with." He continued, "We were asked to drink
water with medicines (or teas) in the appropriate seasons for a reason. They had value and were there to help us maintain our health.
It reminded us that we are a part of the natural world, a part of that
cyclical and changing dynamic."

Gregory Cajete, a leader of the "Native science" movement
explains, "We cannot help but participate with the world. Whether
we acknowledge and are creatively open to the perceptions that will
result, or remain oblivious to its influence and creative possibilities
toward deeper understanding, is our decision. This is the perpetual
trap of Western science and the perpetual dilemma of Western society: all humans are in constant interaction with the physical reality. Western science and society perpetuate the illusion of 'objective'
detachment and psychological disassociation." He further notes,
"Native science continually relates to and speaks of the world as full
of *active* entities with which people engage. Native languages are

verb based, and the words that describe the world emerge directly from actively perceived experience. In a sense language 'choreographs' and/or facilitates the continual orientation of Native thought and perception toward active participation, active imagination, and active engagement with all that makes up the natural reality" (2000, 26-27). He observes, "This active perpetual engagement with the animate world was termed the 'participation mystique' by French anthropologist Lucien Levy-Bruhl to describe the "animistic logic of Indigenous, oral peoples for whom ostensibly 'inanimate' objects like stones or mountains are thought to be alive, and from whom certain names, spoken out loud, may be felt to influence the things or beings that they name, for whom particular plants, particular animals, particular places, persons, and powers may all be felt to 'participate' in one another's existence, influencing each other and being influenced in return" (Cajete 2000, 26-27).

Unfortunately, Western science devalues or discredits this view by often using pejorative terms such as *primitive, mythological,* or *ancestor worship* to describe these beliefs about animism and our dynamic relationship with the world around us. Johnson and Murton (2007) write, "Western people have sought to remove themselves from nature and the 'savage' non-European masses." They see indigenous voices being much needed in "re/placement . . . within constructions of nature and seek to begin healing the disenchantment caused through the rupture between culture and nature in Western science." As we experience more devastation and pollution of natural resources, more corporate takeover of human rights to water, clean air, and land, indigenous peoples are providing us with ancient knowledge systems that call for a greater understanding of how we *all* are connected to each other and we all need to examine our "localness" to what is available around us. We have displaced that local and indigenous knowledge from the reductionist, Western scientific way of seeing the world, and many are now realizing just how critical that is to knowing how to balance, heal, and preserve that which sustains us. This Native science movement is germinating throughout Indian country, but also through those Western-trained scientific disciplines that see the urgency in utilizing these ancient indigenous epistemologies to create a better relationship with the natural world, in such disciplines as environmental health, public health, anthropology, and physics.

One Cherokee elder said, "We have been here for more than 12,000 years observing, measuring, and replicating how we interact with our environment. When we conduct ritual and ceremony, we are using our science to heal us, to provide us with *tohi'* and to take responsibility for our place in this world" (T. B., Cherokee, 2003, pers. comm.). *Tohi'*, a Cherokee concept for well-being has multifaceted definitions relating to health and balance. Belt and Altman (2009) provide an excellent discussion of *tohi'* with examples of how this concept reflects our relationship in the natural world. In a broader discussion of Native science, Dawn Martin-Hill situates Native understanding of the natural world, the cosmos, and how humans fit into these systems as "knowledge [that] is spiritually based and eco-logically derived" (2008, 10). She cites Gregory Cajete's work regarding indigenous epistemologies and reflects on his understanding of how spiritual laws govern the natural world and humans' interrelated existence. She says, "He explores how ethnoscience reflects the uniqueness of place and is thus inherently tied to land and expressed through language and cultural practice," and we would include in that, tied to land and water (Martin-Hill 2008, 9).

Ceremonies and ritual, particularly those using water, are tremendously important. As mentioned previously, elders believe that water carries spirit. The "distinguished physician Deepak Chopra echoes the awe of the paradoxes of spirit: 'The spirit is a real force. It's as real as gravity, it's as real as time. It's equally abstract, equally as incomprehensible and mysterious and difficult to grasp conceptually" (Hammerschlag and Silverman 1997, 9). Dr. Carl Hammerschlag, a former Indian Health Service psychiatrist says, "We believe that true healing requires the participation of one's spiritual self. We believe that stories and ceremonies are the surest ways of touching the human spirit and promoting healing. . . . Science has begun to notice something that healers have always known: Feeling connected to people and things outside yourself helps to keep you healthy and assists you when you're ill" (Hammerschlag and Silverman 1997, 15).

An interesting study by Masaru Emoto has come under scrutiny by some in the Western scientific community. His studies exemplify some of the concepts expressed by elders regarding water, spirit, and the interrelatedness of water with us and all other things. In his book *The True Power of Water* (2003), he set out to record that "water changes in quality according to the information it takes in." Being the first to ever photograph water crystals in 1994, Emoto began to research the Japanese concept of hado, water given good energy. He says that since the human body is 70 percent water, we have a connection to water and an essence related to water that most don't fully understand:

> Water is sensitive to a subtle form of energy called *hado*. It is this form of energy that affects the quality of water and the shape in which water crystals form. All existing things have vibrations, or *hado*. This energy is either positive or negative and is easily transmitted to other existing things. The thought "you fool" carries its own *hado*, which the water absorbs and displays as deformed crystals when frozen. On the other hand, when water is exposed to positive thoughts, beautiful crystals are formed that reflect positive *hado*. *Hado* is integrally woven into

the implications of water's response to our positive or negative energy. (21)

Emoto goes on to examine the shape and nature of water as it is exposed not only to human energy but also to toxins and to explore other contexts of natural water that has been interfered with. His water crystal photographs are striking and convincing.

David Bohm, world renowned physicist, worked with native elders in the last few decades of his life and found that much of Native science was completely in line with his understanding of modern physics. Not only that, but his work with natives such as Blackfoot elder Leroy Little Bear, furthered his own research. For example, his theory of implicate or enfolded order has been understood as part of constructs from his experience with Native ceremony and world-view. "Bohm suggested that, in its deepest essence, reality, or 'that which is,' is not a collection of material objects in interaction but a process or a movement of the whole. The stable forms we see around us are not primary in themselves but only the temporary unfold-ing of the underlying implicate order. To take rocks, trees, plants, or stars as the primary reality would be like assuming that the vortices in a river exist in their own right and are totally independent of the river itself" (Peat 2002, 140).

David Peat, student of Bohm and Little Bear and author of *Blackfoot Physics* (2002), discusses the questions regarding the build-ing blocks of water, molecules of hydrogen and oxygen, and the fact that how they are arranged together is not fully understood. Instead, he explains that their attraction or bond, is one that can involve being "written into." He goes on to say that "the more we think of the human body, not as a machine, or a set of biological reactions, but as the physical manifestation of fields of meaning and processes of information, the more we can be open to the presence of subtle levels of energy, matter, and spirit within healing" (139).

We can hopefully begin to take much longer measure of the Native science that Cherokee and other indigenous peoples hold true. In doing so, we may look upon our most sacred resources, such as water, more seriously and realize its quality and access is critical for everyone, physically, culturally, and spiritually.

Works Cited

Anderson, William L., Jane L. Brown, and Anne F. Rogers, eds. 2010. *The Payne-Butrick Papers*. Lincoln: University of Nebraska Press.

Berry, Wendell. 2005. *Given: Poems*. Berkeley, CA: Counter Point Press.

Binns, Cory. 2012. "How Long Can a Person Survive without Water?" Live Science, November 30. http://www.livescience.com/32320-how-long-can-a-person-survive-without-water.html.

Bohm, David. 1996. *On Dialogue*. New York: Routledge Press.

Cajete, Gregory. 2000. *Native Science: Natural Laws of Interdependence*. Santa Fe, NM: Clear Light Publishers.

Cherokee Nation. 2012. http://www.cherokee.org/AboutTheNation/Culture/General/24405/Information.aspx.

Colorado Water Information. 2013. http://www.waterinfo.org/resources/waterfacts.

Emoto, Masaru. 2003. *The True Power of Water*. New York: ATRIA Books.

Fogelson, Raymond D. 1961. "Change, Persistence, and Accommodation in Cherokee Medico-Magical Beliefs." In *Symposium on Cherokee and Iroquois Culture*, edited by W. N. Fenton and J. Gulick, 215-25. Bureau of American Ethnology Bulletin 180. Washington, DC: Smithsonian Institution.

———. 1962. *The Cherokee Ball Game: A Study in Southeastern Ethnology*. PhD diss., University of Pennsylvania.

———. 2004. *Handbook of North American Indians, Vol. 14, Southeast*. Washington, DC: Smithsonian Institution Press.

Free Drinking Water. 2013. http://www.freedrinkingwater.com/water-education/water-health.htm.

Hammerschlag, Carl A., and Howard D. Silverman. 1997. *Healing Ceremonies*. New York: Berkeley Publishing Group.

Harvard University Pluralism. 2013. http://www.pluralism.org/reports/view/174.

Holland, T. J. 2013. "The Importance of Water to the Cherokee Worldview." Paper Presented at the Annual Meeting of the Southern Anthropological Society, Johnson City, TN.

Jiang, Shan. 2014. "Therapeutic Landscapes and Healing Gardens: A Review of Chinese Literature in the Relation to the Studies in Western Countries." *Frontiers of Architectural Research* 3 (2): 141-53.

Johnson, Jay T., and Brian Murton. 2007. "Re/placing Native Science: Indigenous Voices in Contemporary Constructions of Nature." *Geographical Research* 45 (2): 121-29.

Kilpatrick, Alan Edwin. 1991. "'Going to Water': A Structural Analysis of Cherokee Purification Rituals." *American Indian Culture and Research Journal* 15 (4): 49-58.

Kilpatrick, Jack Frederick, and Anna Gritts Kilpatrick. 1970. "Notebook of a Cherokee Shaman." In *Smithsonian Contributions to Anthropology* 2 (6): 83-125. Washington, DC: Smithsonian Institution Press.

Lefler, Lisa J., ed. 2009. *Under the Rattlesnake: Cherokee Health and Resiliency*. Tuscaloosa: University of Alabama Press.

———. 2012. Fieldnotes. Cherokee, NC.

Martin-Hill, Dawn. 2008. *The Lubicon Lake Nation: Indigenous Knowledge and Power*. Toronto, Canada: University of Toronto Press.

McClinton, Rowena, ed. 2007. *The Moravian Springplace Mission to the Cherokees*. Lincoln: University of Nebraska Press.

Nightingale, Florence. 1860. *Notes on Nursing: What It Is, and What It Is Not*. http://digital.library.upenn.edu/women/ nightingale/nursing/nursing.html

Peat, David F. 2002. *Blackfoot Physics*. Boston, MA: Weiser Books.

Riggs, Brett. 2013. "Petroglyphs of the Cherokee." Paper Presented at the Annual Meeting of the Southern Anthropological Society, Johnson City, TN.

Thomas, Robert K. 1958. "Cherokee Values and Worldview." Unpublished Manuscript. University of North Carolina at Chapel Hill.

The Influences of Vodou on Medical Pluralism and Treatment-Seeking Behavior among Haitian Immigrants in the United States: Suggestions for Cultural Competency Programs

Sarah Hoover

Introduction

Haitian immigrants are highly affected by stigma when they migrate to the United States because of their spiritual practices. This stigmatization has led to some complicated developments in the ways that they transition to life in their new country as transnational communities. The most notable aspects of this transition are the strong ties many of them continue to maintain with Haiti, both physically and spiritually. Transnationals can be defined as migrants who are not completely part of their host society or of the native land from which they come. However, their identities are shaped by both because they continue to remain active in the cultures of each society. Haitian immigrants to the United States fit this description in many ways. This paper will focus on the spiritual ties that numerous Haitians hold with their homeland, the resulting medical pluralism that comes from this spiritual transnationalism, the barriers this can pose to health care for Haitian immigrants, and the ways in which American cultural competency programs need to address these problems.

Medical practitioners in the United States are trained in cultural competency classes to be sensitive to the beliefs and values of people of varying religions, ethnicities, and socioeconomic backgrounds. Haitian immigrants pose a challenge to the competency model in particular because of their unique and stigmatized Vodoun belief system. For example, Americans typically seek biomedical care in the early stages of an illness and prenatal care throughout a pregnancy. However, Haitian patients will not usually consider doing such things because of their beliefs in magic, their reliance on "hot-cold" equilibriums, and their distrust of those outside their circles of family and friends (Phelps 2004). A brief summary of the history of Haitian migration and magical beliefs, will frame my discussion.

A Brief History of Haiti

Haiti occupies the western part of the island of Hispaniola, sharing it with the Dominican Republic to the East. According to Nikki Miller, in her 2000 article, Christopher Columbus arrived on the island in 1492. What followed were years of unrest. As the island became colonized by the Spanish, the Arawak Natives succumbed to disease and mistreatment. This resulted in the import of African slaves, who eventually took control of the country after the French also attempted to settle there. The mixture of cultures and religions resulted in Vodou, which incorporates aspects of French Catholicism and African tribal beliefs. This syncretism is the result of a period of time when Vodou was banned and its followers were able to hide their altars behind images of Catholic saints who eventually took on Vodoun spiritual traits of their own.

In the 1950s, the country experienced political turmoil. The self-declared president-for-life, "Papa Doc" Duvalier, promised to eliminate class disparities that led to the marginalization of rural, black populations. In reality, he inflicted fear and violence on the people of Haiti, causing many to flee the country. The first people to migrate to the United States in 1957 were those who were well educated and had the privilege of mobility. They were the mulattos whose political authority had been challenged by Duvalier. The next wave of immigrants was from the upper-class black population who had realized that Duvalier had not kept his promise to give them influence in society. More recently, other immigrants have arrived and continue to arrive in the United States hoping to escape the extreme poverty and persecution they faced in Haiti. They come looking for better health and economic opportunity, and they bring with them their religious beliefs, which influence every facet of life, especially health care.

Vodou

Vodou is centered on a belief in spirits and ancestors who can be communicated with through religious practitioners such as *houngans* (priests) and *mambos* (priestesses). The spirits, called *loa*, each represent a facet of life, such as the home, family, the harvest, or protection from evil (McCarthy-Brown 1991). For example, Papa Legba is the gatekeeper to the spirit world, meaning that all ceremonies must begin with prayers to him in order to open the gate; Ogoun is a warrior spirit who is called upon for protection; and Damballa-Wedo is a loving father who is credited with creation. Other spirits who deal with small requests and everyday situations are Kouzen and his female counterpart Kouzinn. Ancestors are treated in much the same way as the loa, with elaborate ceremonies, meals, and prayers (McCarthy-Brown 1991, 8)

The loa and ancestors are "fed" at these ceremonies in the hope that they will be pleased and will then grant the requests of the family or community. This demonstrates the importance of reciprocity to the followers of Vodou (Miller 2000). Without reciprocity, the loa or ancestors can become angry and inflict diseases and misfortune, or people can be cursed by a person who is unhappy with them.

Certain ceremonies are conducted to protect people from the evil intentions of others. Predetermined fate is yet another trait of this religion, meaning that those who follow Vodou tend to believe that their fate has been determined since birth. This could dissuade them from seeking medical help for illnesses and injuries that they believe were "meant" to happen and are out of their control (DeSantis 1989).

The loa are communicated with through spirit possession. After praying with the congregation, the houngan or mambo may enter a possession trance and take on the voice, personality, and even physical props of the spirit with whom the people wish to speak. They are then fed food that has been placed on an altar, and dancing and singing usually commence during these ceremonies. The people may request healing or protection, which are administered by the houngan/mambo as herbal preparations, incantations, prayers, and animal sacrifices (Miller 2000). Each of these services has a price, depending on the prices of the supplies needed. It is also believed that these things must be done by a religious practitioner rather than a Western doctor.

Those who follow Vodou believe that there is a distinct division of illness that must be observed (Miller 2000). Some illnesses are natural, caused by forces within the body. These illnesses are thought to be best treated by a Western medical practitioner. However, outside forces are feared and revered in Vodou. Spells, hexes, and curses can affect people's health and well-being, which are at the mercy of another's will, especially if someone is upset with them. If one person does wrong to another, the wrongdoer may then fear that the other person will have a priest or priestess curse them. To counteract the evil will of another person and to treat such a supernatural ailment, only a religious practitioner can be called upon.

Another aspect of Vodou medical beliefs involves the humoral balance of the body (DeSantis 1989; Miller 2000). It is believed that the body must be kept at a hot-cold equilibrium. This is done through the ingestion of foods that are classified as either "hot" or "cold." For example, a new mother is in danger of becoming quickly chilled, which could do damage to herself and her baby. In order to avoid this, the woman is kept in seclusion for a month postpartum and fed only foods that are classified as "hot." If the mother becomes chilled, the resulting disequilibrium can be passed on to the child through breast milk, resulting in tetanus or diarrhea (Miller 2000).

The various practitioners that are called upon in Vodou include houngans and mambos, herbalists, midwives, bonesetters, injectionists, and Western doctors. As mentioned above, the houngan/ mambo treats illnesses classified as supernatural. This means that the illness comes on suddenly and is believed to be caused by a breach of reciprocity between the person and a loa or ancestor, or the illness is sent by another person who is angry or envious. The houngan/ mambo will diagnose illnesses by using cards, cowrie shells, pieces of coconut shell, and/or a possession trance in which they call upon the spirits for assistance.

The herbalist, called *docte fe* or *medsen fey*, meaning "leaf doctor," is consulted for commonplace or natural disorders such as colds, worms, diarrhea, and stomachache. They are also adept at treating *mal dyok*, or evil eye, which is an affliction of young children caused by the envious gaze of another person. It is characterized by symptoms associated with protein-calorie malnutrition.

The midwife delivers most babies in rural areas of Haiti and performs most of the prenatal care. Along with the concern about the hot-cold equilibrium of a mother and child, childbearing women are susceptible to an illness caused by fright or exposure to negative emotions called *move san* that can cause spoiled breast milk, which in turn can negatively affect the infant. Midwives are called upon to deal with all of these maladies and many preventive precautions.

The bonesetter treats broken bones and musculoskeletal or joint discomfort through massage, physical manipulation, poultices, and prayer. The injectionist administers parenteral preparations of herbal or Western medicines.

Barriers to Health Care

The Western physician is usually accessed to provide preventative care. Also, certain illnesses, such as AIDS and tuberculosis, can be either naturally or supernaturally acquired, and therefore can be treated by any of the practitioners, including Western physicians (Miller 2000). However, access to biomedical care when it is needed is a problem for many Vodou-following Haitian immigrants. Along with financial burdens and the general unease that immigrant populations have with using the American health care system, this population must navigate between culturally appropriate remedies and a common distrust of Western physicians.

While Vodou is centered on healing and well-being, the beliefs and practices outlined above can also act as barriers for Haitian immigrants seeking health care in the United States. For all immigrants, lack of familiarity with the American health care system acts as an enormous barrier, preventing those who may not fully understand how to navigate it from seeking care. A primary problem for immigrants is that of undefined residency status. Irregular immigrants might feel that they would be in danger of deportation if they seek medical care from Western institutions.

Mental health care presents a particular problem. In the case of Haitian immigrants, stigma associated with Vodoun beliefs can keep them from seeking treatment. Some studies have shown that there are reports of Vodou followers being diagnosed with a mental illness simply for their beliefs in Vodou (Miller 2000). In addition, Haitian immigrants may believe anything wrong with a person's mental state to be caused by outside, supernatural forces and that it should be treated by a spiritual ceremony or treatment. This prevents a Haitian immigrant who follows Vodou from seeking treatment from a psychologist or psychiatrist.

Haitian immigrants also prefer private care rather than seeking care from public clinics and hospitals (Miller 2000). This is because of distrust, or a belief that public health care is inadequate and can result in humiliation. However, in most cases, private doctors are not affordable for this demographic. This leaves many Haitian immigrants unwilling to seek health care, or they could revert to a home remedy or religious cure.

The above-mentioned Vodou belief in fatalism acts as a barrier as well. The strong belief that a person's fate is predetermined and that whatever befalls a person is meant to be and cannot be helped could lead to less effort in accessing medical care when sick or injured. While this is true, many women will still seek preventative care for their children and continue to try to control a disease once it has shown symptoms, a common practice among Haitian immigrants (Miller 2000).

A final barrier that Haitian immigrants in particular face is associated with HIV/AIDS. According to Glick-Schiller, because of the high rates of HIV in the Haitian population, the waves of Haitian immigrants that made their way to the United States in the mid- and late-1900s were stigmatized. This stigma extends to the present day and might be yet another reason that such immigrants do not seek Western care for fear of humiliation and unequal treatment.

Two barriers in particular stand between Western physicians and their Vodou-following patients. As mentioned above, people can be immediately diagnosed with a mental illness simply because of their belief in Vodou. Many biomedical doctors simply dismiss a person's spiritual beliefs, especially those they are unfamiliar with. Vodou falls into such a category. A dismissal of a person's strong belief system can lead to distrust and noncompliance with medical treatment. These negative and stereotyped views of Vodou and Haitian people need to be addressed and changed. While Miller (2000) insists that showing support for a patient's spirituality encourages a stronger relationship with the patient, she goes on to explain that delving deep into the religion in order to understand it must be an individual decision. This illustrates that Western practitioners do not need to understand every detail of every ritual and spirit, but a basic understanding and respect for the values and beliefs of each patient is needed.

Another barrier is manifested in a simple difference in culture between Americans and many Haitians: that of confidentiality. While Haitian patients have been observed as being shy in the clinic setting, it has also been found that a common practice in Haiti is to involve a person's (especially a child's) family in the diagnosis and treatment of a disease or injury. A Western physician is ethically bound by the law to keep certain medical information private between him and his patient, but this extreme privacy could leave Vodou-following Haitian immigrants feeling secluded and isolated from their own family and friends. The problem of isolation is a pattern with immigrants from all over the world, and feeling alone and at the mercy of a health care system that does not include a person's loved ones can lead many immigrants to decide not to seek care. With the permission of the patient, involving family members in the process may help the physician to gain trust (Miller 2000). This would call for policy changes that could alter rules dictating the number of people allowed to accompany patients during doctor visits, along with confidentiality requirements of doctors who treat individuals who request the involvement of others.

The Importance of Cultural Competency

The following reasons for a "compelling need for cultural competence" are extracted from Cohen and Goode's 1999 policy brief for the *Rationale for Cultural Competence in Primary Care*. The reasons given by this report for an understanding between Western physicians and their immigrant patients are that

> the perception of illness and disease and their causes varies by culture; diverse belief systems exist related to health, mental health, healing, and well-being; culture influences help-seeking behaviors and attitudes toward primary care providers; individual preferences affect traditional and other approaches to primary care; patients must overcome personal experiences of biases within primary care systems; and primary care providers from culturally and linguistically diverse groups are underrepresented in current service delivery systems.

The above reasons apply to the Vodou-following Haitian immigrants. Cohen and Goode continue to argue that to meet these needs, medical policies must respond to demographic changes in the United States, eliminate disparities, improve the quality of services and outcomes, meet accreditation mandates, gain a competitive edge in the marketplace, and decrease liability and malpractice claims by educating physicians, nurses, and even administrative staff through cultural competency training. This would require that organizations

> have a defined set of values and principles, and demonstrate behaviors, attitudes, policies, and structures that enable [medical care providers] to work effectively cross-culturally; have the capacity to (1) value diversity, (2) conduct self-assessment, (3) manage the dynamics of difference, (4) acquire and institutionalize cultural knowledge and (5) adapt to diversity and the cultural contexts

of the communities they serve; [and] incorporate the above in all aspects of policy making, administration, practice/service delivery and involve systematically consumers/families.

It has been well established that the poor treatment of minority groups can lead to poor health outcomes. Therefore, the significance of a cultural competency program would be to improve patient compliance and health outcomes, to incorporate the voices of marginalized populations in their health care, and to find common ground between health care providers and patients. The purpose of cultural competence is to train providers to deliver services appropriate to various cultural backgrounds, and the development of such a program requires research gathered by medical anthropologists that can inform curriculum, increase awareness, and enhance practitioner capacity building.

Pulling it All Together

As demonstrated by the preceding description of the beliefs of Vodou and the stigmas that Haitian immigrants in general face in the United States, there is a great need for understanding between Western doctors and this particular demographic. Adopted largely from Miller (2000), the following is a detailed list of changes that can be made in the doctor-patient relationship that can result in higher compliance and better health outcomes:

First, when treating any recent immigrant, the physician must consider particular problems that affect such groups of people. Because Haiti is an extremely impoverished country, malnutrition is one issue that must be addressed during a first doctor visit. Another issue is that of immunization, which is not a common practice in the rural areas of the country. Therefore, when presented with a recent Haitian immigrant, these two topics must be covered and dealt with.

The doctor will need to administer the appropriate immunizations, especially to children, and treat any signs of malnutrition displayed by the patient. Another important step will be to make a dental referral, because numerous rural Haitian immigrants have never seen a dentist before. As is the common paradox for any group of rural immigrants to the United States, their dental health may decline due to the introduction of sugary, processed foods and their unfamiliarity with dental visits.

Second, as DeSantis described in her 1989 study of Haitian and Cuban mothers and their children, an understanding of the Haitian cultural view of the body is essential. When DeSantis interviewed mothers about the various symptoms their children show during illness,

> the Haitian mothers gave global descriptions of the child's experience, such as "the child looks very sick;" "he looks very bad;" "it (fever) dries up the body;" it "bring on other things;" the "child does not develop normally;" it makes him "very sick;" and the child looks "sick and fragile."

She also says that, due to the belief that the entire body is implicated when symptoms appear, Haitian immigrants will most likely describe their ailment or illness in terms of their entire body, rather than isolating the affected part of the body. Therefore, the physician needs to be aware of how patients perceive a treatment in terms of their cultural beliefs about the body as a whole. To establish common ground, the physician should describe its effects on the entire body, rather than focusing on one particular area. This could result in higher compliance with the treatment, since the patients will better understand the treatment's purpose in terms of the entire body. Also, certain parts of the body should not be uncovered due to moral beliefs, so to prevent offending the patient, asking them to disrobe should be avoided or dealt with in a sensitive manner (Phelps 2004).

A third, very important, step would be an initial screening for venereal diseases and HIV, considering the high rates of such diseases among this population. However, the act of suggesting this screening needs to be done with sensitivity because of the stigmas described above. It might be important to make it clear that the suggestion is being made not because of the person's race or ethnicity but because it is a beneficial procedure that all immigrants, and all people for that matter, should go through.

Along with being sensitive toward stigmas associated with the population of Haitian immigrants in general, a physician needs to show understanding in terms of religious beliefs. Showing respect and remaining nonjudgmental about spiritual beliefs and ethno-medical practices associated with Vodou can help build friendship and trust between doctor and patient. Medical pluralism can be fostered by understanding why patients seek care other than Western biomedicine and how exactly their remedies and ceremonies work.

Last, maintaining this trusting relationship and including the patient's input and their family's input is the best way to reach a point of understanding. However, this approach has its challenges and limits. Most doctors, other than private care physicians, have only a limited amount of time with each patient, resulting in little or no relationship established. In order for this to change, policies regarding time management and the numbers of patients seen in the course of a day need to change. Also, patient confidentiality is taken extremely seriously in the United States, and physicians may fear that including the input of people other than the patient will result in breeches of this confidentiality. These issues need to be fully discussed with patients in order include their input and gain their permission to embrace the participation of their family.

Discussion and Conclusion

Haitian immigrants, especially those who prescribe to beliefs of the religion of Vodou, have been stigmatized in the United States for decades. Not only has the stigma of high rates of HIV/AIDS among Haitian groups affected the health-seeking behaviors of this community, but stigmas associated with spiritual beliefs have also made communication and understanding between doctors and Haitian patients difficult. On top of this, the religion of Vodou and its associated beliefs about fatalism, the body, medicine, and traditional remedies act as barriers to health care themselves. As demonstrated in this paper, Haitian immigrants, especially those who follow Vodou, face a mountain of challenges that can prevent them from receiving much-needed health care. As one author phrases the problem,

> the identity of Haitian immigrants is being forged in the complex and sometimes conflicting relationship between their historical experiences as members of subordinate populations, their cultural backgrounds, their continuing ties to their home societies, and the conditions, structures, and ideologies of the dominant capitalist societies in which they have settled. (Glick-Schiller 1990)

Vodou-following Haitian immigrants tend to separate illness and disease into two categories: natural and supernatural. Depending on the categorization of a disease, the individual will seek out either a religious practitioner or a Western physician. This, along with fear of persecution and deportation, stigma associated with HIV/AIDS, a common preference for expensive private care, beliefs about mental health and fatalism, and other traits, can form barriers to health care and result in undesirable health outcomes. Therefore, it would be important for American doctors, nurses, and administrative medical staff who treat such patients to be trained in their history and belief system to an extent that they can communicate in a culturally sensitive manner.

However, many cultural competency programs have proven to foster racism and stereotypes that result in little or no improvement in the treatment of patients from diverse religious, ethnic, and socioeconomic backgrounds. A new model of cultural competency is greatly needed to address Haitian immigrants. One way to do this could be to employ participatory action research by distributing surveys, conducting interviews with both health care workers and Haitian patients, and conducting participant observation in health care facilities. This would allow an even greater, in-depth look into the needs of this population and the barriers they face when seeking health care. It could also lead to a better understanding of the relationship between Western physicians and Haitian patients.

Based on the findings, an updated model of cultural competency training could be developed and established in American health care. This program could be more holistic and comprehensive, allowing health workers to learn about the complex history and religion that influences the decisions of Haitian immigrants. It could break down barriers and do away with harmful racism, stereotypes, and stigma, allowing for better access to health care. The ultimate goal would be to improve physician sensitivity to differing cultures in general, along with improving patient compliance and health outcomes in this population.

Another suggestion would be a possible collaboration attempt between Vodou religious practitioners and biomedical doctors. As is explained above, Vodou-following Haitian immigrants have a wealth of traditional healers on whom they can call for the treatment of various maladies. Perhaps if a program were created that could bring these healers into close contact with biomedical practitioners, a better understanding could be born between them. While this may be a far-fetched idea in American society where doctors hold the ultimate authoritative knowledge and are unlikely to accept alternate forms of healing, it could be possible in the coming years as globalization further unites all corners of the world. A program such as this could also create networks of referrals between the differing cultures, allowing Haitian immigrants to navigate more easily between their two worlds.

It is obvious that there are major divides between Vodou and biomedicine, leaving Vodou-following Haitian immigrants in the United States to fall through the cracks. With an improved system of cultural competency training resulting from the input of the Haitian immigrant community, these divides can be crossed, and cooperation between the two cultures can be established. With the ultimate goal being better health outcomes for immigrants, physicians need to be trained to be culturally sensitive, to shed their judgmental opinions about other healing practices, and to effectively communicate with Haitian patients. To conclude, as Miller (2000) puts it, "It is clear that to provide culturally acceptable care for this population, we must both increase our understanding of their belief system and rid ourselves of the distorted way this culture and belief system are viewed. . . . The health care provider can also achieve success by offering nonjudgmental suggestions about health conditions that the patient prefers to treat through an ethnomedical system or a combination of ethnomedicine and biomedicine, by establishing and maintaining a good therapeutic relationship, and by hoping for the best."

Works Cited

Cohen, E., and Goode, T. D. 1999. *Rationale for Cultural Competence in Primary Health Care.* Policy Brief No. 1. Washington, DC: National Center for Cultural Competence.

Colin, Jessie. 2010. Cultural and Clinical Care for Haitians PowerPoint presentation, http://www.state.in.us/isdh/files/ Haiti_Cultural_and_Clinical_Care_Presentation_Read-Only.pdf.

DeSantis, L. 1989. "Health Care Orientations of Cuban and Haitian Immigrant Mothers: Implications for Health Care Professionals." *Medical Anthropology* 12 (1): 69-89.

Glick-Schiller, N. 1990. "Everywhere We Go, We Are in Danger": Ti Manno and the Emergence of a Haitian Transnational Identity." *American Ethnologist* 17 (2): 329-47.

McCarthy-Brown, K. 1991. *Mama Lola.* Berkeley: University of California Press.

Miller, N. 2000. "Haitian Ethnomedical Systems and Biomedical Practitioners: Directions for Clinicians." *Journal of Transcultural Nursing* 11 (3): 204-11.

Phelps, L. 2004. Cultural Competency, Haitian Immigrants, and Rural Sussex County, Delaware, http://www.salisbury.edu/ nursing/haitiancultcomp/default.htm.

About the Contributors

LESLY-MARIE BUER is a doctorial candidate in the Department of Anthropology at the University of Kentucky. She holds a graduate certificate in Gender and Women's Studies from the University of Kentucky. Her primary research interests include women's health, substance abuse, and women's lived experiences in Appalachia.

ANTHONY P. CAVENDER is a Professor of Anthropology at East Tennessee State University. He specializes in the study of ethnomedicine and has conducted research in the highlands of Ecuador, Southern Appalachia, and Zimbabwe. He is the author of *Folk Medicine in Southern Appalachia* (2003, University of North Carolina Press) and coeditor of *A Tennessee Folklore Sampler* (2009, The University of Tennessee Press).

LISA CURTIN is a Professor of Psychology at Appalachian State University. She conducts research on rural mental health service delivery.

BRIAN HOEY is an Associate Professor of Anthropology in the Department of Sociology & Anthropology at Marshall University. He received his BA in Human Ecology from the College of the Atlantic and PhD in Anthropology from the University of Michigan. His ethnographic research explores the social, cultural, and personal impacts of economic restructuring through the lens of community, development, and phenomenon of lifestyle migration. In addition to a continuing interest in career change, identity, and the moral meanings of work, Hoey has a longstanding interest in the anthropology of space and place and, in particular, the effects of built environments on human health. Hoey has published on these and other subjects in the *American Ethnologist, City and Society, Journal of Anthropological Research, Journal of Contemporary Ethnography, Journal of Contemporary Ethnography, Ethnology,* and several book chapters, and his book *Opting for Elsewhere* (2014, Vanderbilt University Press).

SARAH HOOVER is a native of Jonesborough, Tennessee. She earned her bachelor's degree in cultural anthropology from East Tennessee State University in 2012 and her master's degree in applied medical anthropology from the University of Memphis in 2014. Sarah now works in Knoxville, Tennessee, as a Research and Evaluation Assistant with the Amputee Coalition.

SUSAN E. KEEFE is a Professor of Anthropology at Appalachian State University. She is editor of *Appalachian Cultural Competency: A Guide for Medical, Mental Health and Social Service Professionals* (2005, University of Tennessee Press) and *Participatory Development in Appalachia: Cultural Identity, Community, and Sustainability* (2009, University of Tennessee Press).

LINDSEY KING is an Assistant Professor of Anthropology at East Tennessee State University. Her research focuses on material culture and most recently the material traditions found in religious pilgrimage. She is the author of *Spiritual Currency in Northeast Brazil* (2014, University of New Mexico Press).

LISA J. LEFLER is a Medical Anthropologist and received her PhD from The University of Tennessee, Knoxville, in 1966. She is currently Director of Culturally Based Native Health Programs at Western Carolina University and is founder and Executive Director of the Center for Native Health, Inc.

JAMES C. TOLLESON was born in San Rafael, California, and grew up in Hendersonville, located in the mountains of western North Carolina. He graduated from Davidson College (NC) in 2013 with a BA in Ethnic Studies. His degree focused on environmental justice, education, and United States social history. Other formative experiences include working with the Children's Defense Fund's Freedom Schools Program, learning about the effects of poverty, mass incarceration, and health inequity on young people growing up in the United States. In Detroit, he worked with the Feedom Freedom Growers to understand how the urban agriculture movement addressed food insecurity in historically underresourced African American neighborhoods and promoted a vision of rebuilding the city with justice and sustainability. Currently, he works with an organization called FoodCorps in Greenwood, Mississippi, where he has enjoyed building school gardens, working with young people, and learning more about building a community movement for food justice and health.